Needs Gap

Simple Guide to Manage Autoimmune Disease and Chronic Pain- Including Fun Recipes

Pantea Kalhor

Reed Davis, Kellie Lupsha, Tsao-Lin Moy, Betty Khalili, Heather Gray

ACECHOICE PUBLISHING & BRANDING

https://acechoiceidea.com

Copyright

Needs Gap

ISBN-13: 978-1-7780351-4-2

https://acechoiceidea.com

AceChoice Publishing and Branding

Table of Contents

This Book is Dedicated to v

Don't Forget Our Freebies vi

Disclaimer vii

Foreword by Kellie Lupsha, Women's Longevity Expert viii

Editorial Review xi

Praise for Needs Gap xii

Introduction 1

CHAPTER 1: Functional Labs and How They Can Help 4

By Reed Davis, Founder of FDN, Board-certified Holistic Health Practitioner (HHP), and Expert in Functional Lab Testing and Natural Protocols 4

CHAPTER 2: Find Your Triggers 22

By Pantea Kalhor, Publisher, Five Times Bestselling Author, FDN Practitioner, Certified Fertility and PTSD Coach 22

CHAPTER 3: Treating Autoimmune Disease with Chinese Medicine 50

By Tsao-Lin Moy, Licensed Acupuncturist, Traditional Chinese Medicine Practitioner, and Herbalist 50

CHAPTER 4: Hidden Causes of Autoimmunity 77

By Heather Gray, FDN Practitioner 77

CHAPTER 5: The Secrets of Longevity; Can We Control Our DNA? 93

By Kellie Lupsha, Women's Longevity Expert 93

CHAPTER 6: How A Little Change in My Mom's Lifestyle Saved Her Life 117

By Betty Khalili, Registered Nurse, and Bestselling Author 117

CHAPTER 7: Some Fun and Healthy Recipes 127

Filet and Veggies by Reed Davis 128

Fruity Breakfast by Pantea Kalhor 131

Home-Made Almond Milk by Tsao-Lin Moy 134
Turkey PHO Grain-free Noodle Soup by Heather Gray 135
Cinnamon Chia Seed Pudding and Breakfast Cookies by Kellie Lupsha 138
Apple Sour Cherry Stew by Betty Khalili 141
Appendix - by Kellie Lupsha 146
Epilogue by Pantea Kalhor 160
About the Authors 162
Pantea Kalhor 163
Reed Davis 166
Tsao-Lin Moy, Bestselling Author, Licensed Acupuncturist, Traditional Chinese Medicine Practitioner, and Herbalist 168
Heather Gray, FDN Practitioner, Lyme Boss 169
Kellie Lupsha, Women's Longevity Expert 171
Betty Khalili, Registered Nurse and Bestselling Author 173

This Book is Dedicated to

Those who care for their health and are tired of being stuck in a cycle of trial and error.

Pantea Kalhor Nov 12, 2022

Don't Forget Our Freebies and Needs Gap Master Class Series. Click Below:

https://acechoiceidea.com/funnel/needs-gap/

Other Books by Pantea Kalhor

1. *Rules of Change for the Better: Real Stories and Your Guide to Tune-Up Your Mood and Transform Your Life to Reach Your Biggest Dreams*
   https://therulesofchange.com

2. *Naturally Conceived: How to Get Pregnant, Explain Unexplained Infertility and Prevent Miscarriages by Unleashing Your Reproductive Power Even Over 40!*
   https://panteakalhor.com

3. *PTSD Compass: Navigate Trauma to Triumph and Renew Your Life*
   https://acechoiceidea.com/funnel/ptsd-compass

4. *The Gap: Simple Steps to Reclaim Your Health and Reverse Most Chronic Diseases*
   https://acechoiceidea.com/funnel/the-gap

Disclaimer

Needs Gap is the collective work of healthcare practitioners. They have shared their solutions in treating their own health crisis or what has worked for them in treating their patients.

The book has been written for educational purposes. The authors and publisher do not intend to diagnose, cure, treat, or prevent any condition or disease. Before you begin any healthcare program, or change your lifestyle, you should consult your physician or another licensed healthcare practitioner to choose the right tool.

This book is not intended as a substitute for consultation with a licensed healthcare practitioner, such as your physician.

Needs Gap provides content related to physical and/or mental health issues. As such, use of this book implies your acceptance of this disclaimer.

Foreword by Kellie Lupsha, Women's Longevity Expert

Being in the healthcare field for over 25 years, I've seen the evolution in mindset from 'the doctors know all' to 'I am in control of my health.' However, as a society, most people, including medical professions, still believe I'll wait until I'm sick and then my doctors will help me. I began my career as a traditionally trained physical therapist from the Mayo Clinic. I was intimately involved with patients experiencing life-threatening illness and injuries. It was a blessing to be a part of this incredible institution and help so many people.

As I continued in my career, I realized most of us in healthcare were only helping people after they were sick, and I was so puzzled as to where is the missing pieces were to help people stay well. I began seeing clients sicker and sicker than well as younger and younger with serious conditions such as stroke, neurological diseases, autoimmune, metabolic disorders, cancer and more. I knew this was not where I wanted to be headed in medicine and healthcare as a practitioner. I also felt a burning desire to be a part of changing this paradigm of just accepting people getting sicker.

I went on a quest to find more about wellness. What I found was exciting, renewing, hopeful and overall delightful was that we, as healthcare practitioners, as well as individuals, can move from the path of illness to wellness. I also found many practitioners, like myself, in search of helping people heal more naturally, teaching clients to stay well, implement lifestyle changes both for physical, mental, and emotional wellbeing. It was here on my journey I met Pantea.

I am blessed to have met Pantea as well as so many other clinicians and wellness experts with a common goal. We are breaking away from sick care to truly apply health and wellness care. There are so many gaps in our current healthcare system and collectively we are shedding light a variety of areas to serve more. We know people are out there begging on their knees for solutions, as well as practitioners looking for solutions to serve their clients more. Pantea is driven to provide a place with her books, podcasts and more to elevate this conversation of the Needs Gap in our community of health for everyone.

We are in a unique time that technology is at our fingertips to learn and share information at the speed of light. Individuals looking for help can search and find lots of solutions. At the same time, technology is advancing so fast doctors, medical providers and all healthcare practitioners struggle to keep up. What is taught in school is almost already old information by the time we are in the world practicing. Therefore, individuals who take an interest in their health can already have elevated conversations with their providers, however because of the tremendous amount of information, as well as how fast technology is changing, it is almost impossible for medical providers to keep up.

With that said, we can't keep blaming our current medical model for the stagnation of our healthcare. Many of us, like the authors of this book, have decided we can help. We do not have to wait for the system to change to help more people. It is sad to see how sick our communities have become under our current model. I am sure each one of us has experienced a loved one, friend or even ourselves who has become very sick or ill and struggling for answers. Most of the current answers given are in the form of medication instead of helping to address the root cause. We have all seen chronic disease on the rise, with so many underlying causes, things we can address every day with different diet and lifestyle choices.

I am proud to be a part of a wellness community of practitioners beginning to change this paradigm. We are teaching people they can and should become the CEO of their health. Teaching people to appreciate their body, mind and soul as it is the most precious gift we have. Unlike a pair of shoes, a car or house that we can trade it or just get a new one when it breaks down, we only have one beautiful body, mind and soul that needs to be nourish, cared for and treated like the precious gift it is.

While we still have many Gaps in our current system, by putting out resources like this book, we are taking steps in making the gaps smaller and smaller for people so everyone can begin to live a life in elevated health as we move from sick care to truly healthcare.

Kellie Lupsha, Women's Longevity Expert

Editorial Review

This book was a true pleasure to edit. Ms. Kalhor and her contributors, while acknowledging the utility of traditional Western medicine for treating certain conditions, gently brought light to some of the areas where Western medicine needs improvement, particularly with regard to chronic illnesses.

Throughout the book, the author and her contributors offered solid, evidence-based alternative treatments for chronic conditions, ranging from thyroid-based disorders to Lyme disease and many others. They provided detailed explanations of their methods, from dietary changes and Functional Diagnostic Nutrition to acupuncture/acupressure and described how and why these methods work.

Best of all, they gave preliminary ideas for readers to try which would not necessarily require going to new healthcare providers or undergoing additional laboratory work right away if the readers aren't in a position to do so. One contributor gave a basic starting point for acupressure that can be done at home, and all of them included healthy recipes that look absolutely delightful. I intend to try some of them myself, just to enjoy the new flavor combinations described!

Elain Roughton

Praise for Needs Gap

DNA traits are not set in Stone as previously taught

This is a must read for anyone with chronic disease or chronic pain who thought that they did not have any further solutions or avenues to pursue. Great to learn that your DNA code may be set, however how it displayed in your body and life is modifiable and we can control that to increase to decrease the good or bad aspects.

Understand your body as a whole system, not just the presenting symptoms

If you struggle with health issues that, no matter how many doctors you visit, you can't resolve, this inspiring book will give you hope. As the author says, "Knowing your body and discovering the root cause helps you find the missing piece of your health issue puzzle". This book helps you understand your body as a whole system, not just as the presenting symptoms. It covers your body systems, functional testing, lifestyle, Chinese medicine and more.

Take charge and become the boss of your health

Great book to give hope for others burdened with health issues and getting no solutions from the health care system. Also, quick reference for tools to take charge of your health.

This book is awesome!!

All the authors had incredible things to say. I learned so much, and the recipes in the end are awesome. I have a few friends with Lyme and autoimmune stuff. I will be getting this book for them! So much practical advice in one book. Truly inspiring.

Very informative and easy to understand

Enjoyed reading the book and tips for improved health & wellness. The folks come from a place of having gone through difficult health issues and "practice what they preach." Easy to understand and written in a clear format. Great book for how to improve your life and health.

What a wonderful, straightforward approach to improving your health.

A super simple read that can help anyone improve their health span. Whether you are dealing with an autoimmune issue or just want to stay as healthy as possible for as long as you can. This is a great place to start or even continue your health journey.

Wonderfully easy read!!

So much information outside the box. Easy to follow help.

Great resource for improving your quality of life!

If you are like me, you are probably wondering how in the world you can manage autoimmune disease and chronic pain. I was so excited when I came across Needs Gap: Simple Guide to Manage Autoimmune Disease and Chronic Pain. This helpful guide provides users with everything they need to know in order to manage their chronic conditions. The book is easy to read and provides users with a wealth of information, including recipes that are perfect for anyone on a restricted diet.

I highly recommend this book to anyone who is struggling to manage their autoimmune disease or chronic pain. It is an essential resource that will help you to improve your quality of life.

Great Guide for Autoimmune & Mystery Illness Sufferers

An easy read, this book covers the secrets behind autoimmune, chronic pain and mystery illness that your doctor will never tell you! Topics cover functional labs, causes and triggers for disease, longevity, genomics, and personalized medicine.

Must read for anyone with autoimmunity that wants to take their power back!

This is a must read for anyone with chronic disease and chronic pain who has gotten lost in the current health care paradigm. Learn from clinicians and their stories who have been in situations that may be similar to yours and find hope for healing and for transformation into the next chapter of a pain free life!

Introduction

Why Did I Write This Book?

Witnessing my aunt who died from cancer in her early forties initiated some strong curiosity in me. I became more interested in learning how to become more immune to chronic pain and fatal disease. I was the advocate of sports competition during school years and always took leaps in participating in swimming, table tennis, running, and jumping competitions. I knew body movement, keeping my weight in a normal range, and following an organic diet could support my health goals. I never imagined that one day I would have to fight with asthma or struggle to have a baby. I thought that because of my lifestyle I wouldn't have health challenges. That might resonate with many of you who read this book. I started a YouTube channel to introduce the power of integrative medicine by interviewing healthcare practitioners who are real-life examples of hope and healing. Then I continued my journey by writing books and educating myself with FDN (Functional Diagnostic Nutrition), fertility coaching, and PTSD (Post Traumatic Stress Disorder) courses to be able to help others who struggle with health issues.

Who Should Read This Book?

If you are suffering from chronic pain such as stomach discomfort, muscle, or back pain and you are stuck in an unlimited cycle of trial and error, then you are in a right place.

If you have been referred to specialists and taken pills to kill your pain but the pain comes back again, I encourage you read this book until the end.

If your stomach hurts whenever you eat something and you need to consume pills to kill your heartburn, then keep reading.

If you have tried different diets but still suffer from weight gain, then I encourage you to carefully flip the pages and write notes while reading.

But if you don't believe in holistic medicine and are not interested in discovering the root cause of your issue, then you really don't need to waste your time by flipping another page.

I used to take Tums pills after each meal. I thought that was normal but discovering the imbalances in my body helped me have delightful meals without worrying about heartburn.

The first time I heard about holistic medicine and changed my lifestyle based on what I learned and studied, I could easily come

back to my ideal weight without even trying to lose weight or follow a strict commercial diet program.

Having constant pain, nail deformation, dark shadows under your eyes, joint pain, or being tired most of the time are not normal. They shouldn't be part of your life. You were born to live a happy, healthy life.

This book is a small yet valuable portion of all my interviews in over 200 episodes on my YouTube channel. It is also part of a master class out of interviews with the authors of this book. They are all accredited and highly respected professionals who dedicate their lives to saving others. They all believe in mind-body connection and holistic medicine. I hope these stories and solutions help you find your own customized health plan and show you the real value of integrative medicine.

Pantea Kalhor

CHAPTER 1: Functional Labs and How They Can Help

By Reed Davis, Founder of FDN, Board-certified Holistic Health Practitioner (HHP), and Expert in Functional Lab Testing and Natural Protocols

I was in the grocery store, about to check out, when someone else in line casually said hello and ended up asking me, "What do you do?" Not wanting to appear anti-social, I decided to answer. But it's hard to put the answer into one phrase when you have a creative mind that constantly races ahead at 20 times the speed of your mouth. This is especially true when having to change concepts quickly. Going from, "What should I bring home for dinner?" to answering, "What do you do?" may not seem like a big challenge to most people. But for others, it may require a shift in gears demanding all manner of self-reflection, consideration of the social effects, and contemplation of life itself!

After a conscious decision to be "social" and provide an adequate and accurate reply, pictures of my daily, weekly, and monthly tasks and activities flew past almost at once. "What do I do?" you ask. My color-coded, on-screen calendar flashed by, listing every kind of meeting and event required to oversee an organization with 35 employees, hundreds of current students, and an active alumnus of over 3000 practitioners in about 50 countries. What do I do? I thought of the managers and team members involved as their faces and voices came into and out of view. I pictured making coffee from 4:30 to 5:00 a.m. almost every day and working at my desk until noon or so, tending to all of that and the 40-plus folders on my desktop.

I saw myself in the gym for an hour before heading onto my property for landscaping and gardening chores and the heavenly "grounding" they provide, especially when driving my tractor and enjoying the amazing view of the lake and mountains in my backyard. What do I do? I saw several piles of books to be read and the infrared sauna calling out to me. A glimpse of the motorcycle collection in my garage slipped by and I wondered *when* the next time is that my wife and I will go for a ride. I thought of my son and started feeling guilty for not visiting him more often and learning to wake-surf on his new boat, and for not spending more time with my wife (unless we're cooking dinner together). Having thus circled back to my present circumstance, I offered up, "Uh, I'm a teacher."

I probably look like a high school math or English teacher, or maybe a college professor, so I was hoping I'd satisfied the inquirer. Don't get me wrong, I love people and socializing and I'm proud of what I do, but I just wanted to check out my groceries and get home to my wife so we could get some dinner going. We both engage in "Time Restricted Eating (TRE)" so when it's time to eat, it's time to eat. Plus, eating organic, dairy-free, gluten-free, real food requires prep time, so I had to get home. Simultaneously, other possible answers were still swirling around in my head. I could have said, "I'm the Founder of Functional Diagnostic Nutrition® (FDN)," or, "I'm the President and CEO of The FDN Certification Course and Community," and more.

Maybe I should have answered, "trash collector" and that would have been the end of it. Too late! I realized I'd set myself up, and sure enough, the next obvious engagement from my curious new grocery line friend was, "Oh. What do you teach?" And he really seemed interested!

My brain went into an even higher gear, or that's what it felt like. I usually get off on it, and I've been told by some interviewers, "Boy, you're good on your feet." But I knew not to go off into a stream of consciousness, dissertation, or story-telling episode. While maintaining a solid social exterior, I considered the enormous amount of anatomy, physiology, and biochemistry that goes into my courses. The ten years of practical experience that are woven into each lesson passed by as I pondered an appropriate short answer. I spent a decade working in a busy clinic before ever teaching my first class. Many of the incredible experiences I had, reviewing thousands of labs, helping thousands of patients by explaining the underlying causes of their health problems popped up, rapid-fire, into my mind.

What do I teach? I thought, "No matter how I answer, it won't even come close to revealing the amount of education, knowledge, skills, and transformation provided by the FDN Certification Course." The FDN Course is experiential, full of practical exercises that guide trainees on their own health journey. As they study the FDN point of view and methodology, trainees learn how to apply it to others as a profession. FDN is not just something you learn about, it's something you must "get." Included in the tuition, all trainees run five functional lab tests on themselves. As they progress through the program, everyone receives several private, one-on-one health coaching sessions to go over their unique results and recommendations. Later, they get to model this behavior and coaching style with mock-up clients.

The goal of the FDN Course is to transform health seekers, health coaches, and allied health practitioners into functional lab experts and exceptional health detectives. By taking a personal journey through the discovery and healing processes, they become effective health-transformation tutors so they can help others on a very deep level.

The lab reports we obtain for clients who submit saliva, urine, blood spot, and stool specimens are used to identify "healing opportunities" and are correlated with problems being experienced by that person. Thus, we help put control of one's health into one's own hands where it belongs. Our trainees (and FDN clients) recognize, "That's not how my regular doctor works."

That's because we don't often use the same tests as "regular doctors," and when we do, we don't review them in the same light. We don't diagnose or treat anything specifically. We know that when a doctor lays down a "diagnosis," he or she is likely leaving a lot of information on the table. In fact, once a client receives a diagnosis, she is likely to be ignoring a plethora of other important areas.

Instead of diagnosing and treating one thing specifically, our labs and lab reports help each client to self-treat everything, non-specifically. That means every cell, tissue, organ, and system — the entire organism — is improved simultaneously!

Case Study

Let me give you an example. Remember, I worked in a wellness center for 10 years, getting invaluable clinical experience before I ever taught my first class. The FDN Course is based on the patterns I recognized and health building principles I discovered while reviewing thousands of lab reports for thousands of people. While I had great mentorship from doctors and lab technicians, I also made my own observations about who got better and who didn't. According to the lab companies I worked with, the sheer volume of lab testing coming from my small office was incredible. One lab director told me I was doing as much lab work as any five doctors combined.

In one case, a woman we'll call Susan was coming into the office for chiropractic care, myofascial release, and some nutrition counseling. This was during the early days when I was solidifying my position as the health director and case manager at the wellness center and only just learning about functional lab work. As such, I greeted many patients in the waiting room and walked them back to a treatment room.

One day, Susan, who we'd been seeing for a few weeks, came in and I could tell she was very unhappy. I said, "Hi, Susan, what's going on today?" As we walked down the hall, her reply was in line with her facial expression. Head down, gazing at the floor, she said,

"Reed, I'm just so tired of regular doctors. All they ever do is give you pills. And this extra 40 pounds I'm carrying around is really frustrating, and it's all because of medication I'm taking for the *hives*." Before I could get a word out, she continued, "I've been on (the med) for two years and the weight just keeps getting worse. And when I went to the doctor for a checkup the other day, I told him how frustrating the weight gain is, and he told me, '*Susan, you have a choice. You can be fat, or you can have the hives.*'" Turning her head towards me now, I could see the tears welling as she continued, "And, Reed, when I told him how depressing that is, he said, 'Well, I'll be happy to write you a prescription for anti-depressants if you like!' So, I'm just so frustrated and miserable."

Now, standing next to a treatment table, she was obviously distraught. She was staring at the floor, looking like she was about to cry. For my part, bedside manner be damned, I blurted out, "Susan, why haven't you tried to determine WHY you get the hives?" Well, let me tell you, her head snapped to attention so hard I thought she wouldn't need her chiropractic adjustment that day!

Obviously, she was very interested. We got her the right tests, went over the results and, to her delight, she was able to get completely off her meds within 9 days. Within two more weeks she was working out to a sweat and taking hot showers, something she revealed she had not done in two years because even on the meds, those activities gave her the hives. Amazing, right? There is nothing like success to make everyone happy, and while individual results may vary, this experience let me know I was on the right track.

Back in the grocery store check-out line, I finally remembered my 15-second elevator speech! As I hurriedly put my credit card into the terminal, I said slowly and clearly, "I teach allied health practitioners how to use functional laboratory work to identify the real, underlying causes of health problems, and all-natural, drug-free, self-directed solutions so they get the best results for themselves and their clients." To his credit, the inquirer gave me a knowing look and nod, and let me exit in peace.

So Simple, Even I Can Understand It!

As I drove home, I wondered if the acknowledgment I received was sincere, or maybe the inquirer was just being polite. In any case, I felt I'd explained my job and my purpose without making it too complicated. I've spent over two decades studying what can be difficult material and making it so that everyone can grasp the meaning. I mean this with all sincerity: "I have to make things so simple that even I can understand it."

In FDN, our view of the health space usually starts with a 30,000-foot view of the entire landscape. Health is our birthright. Our bodies endeavor to survive naturally by way of innate intelligence.

You don't have to teach any cells or organs what their job is. Health depends on one's genetics plus all the *signaling* received, positive or negative, from our diets, the environment, sustained thoughts and emotions, personal habits, and lifestyle or what's known as the "epigenome." The net result is a level of balance and resiliency one could call "health and well-being."

When our state of health drops below a certain threshold, while the body struggles to maintain homeostasis, symptoms finally occur. Symptoms are the last thing to occur in a disease process. In FDN land, we seek to understand why, where is this coming from? Using carefully chosen *functional lab work*, our goal is to identify an entire constellation of *healing opportunities* and use the data to guide behaviors and lifestyle that will restore balance and resiliency.

We do not run one test based on what the problem "sounds like" and hope we guessed right. We do not single out one or two "out of range" lab markers on a report and give it a label, or diagnosis, to be treated specifically. Instead, we run a series of lab work that looks at the most common underlying causes of most chronic degenerative conditions. Again, we look for a whole constellation of healing opportunities that correlate highly with our client's ailments or complaints. The most important consideration for an FDN Practitioner is, "Whose test results are these?" In this chapter, we will only describe the most foundational labs.

Once we have identified multiple healing opportunities, we have our client apply principles of healing that lead to far superior outcomes compared to the diagnosis and treatment model. This approach supports the client, putting them in charge of their health instead of relying on others. I discovered a pattern two decades ago that got the best results. I call that pattern "H-I-D-D-E-N" – the hidden stressors and dysfunctions, sometimes found far upstream from where the disease process is manifesting.

"H-I-D-D-E-N" stands for Hormone, Immune, Digestion, Detoxification, Energy production, and Nervous system balance. We investigate these six areas to identify healing opportunities, discover what is out of balance and what needs to be repaired, rebuilt, or restored to normal functionality.

By first looking into these six areas, plus oxidative stress, and only then applying general principles of health building to every cell, tissue, organ and system, one can heal almost any chronic, downward-spiraling, stress-related condition. People don't come to *us* for broken bones or gunshot wounds or cancerous growths; those require immediate medical attention. It is everything else. It's all the chronic ills of modern living such as chronic fatigue, blood sugar, sleeplessness, chronic inflammation, bad skin, achiness, and even headaches, migraines, and digestive problems.

I'd love to share all the things I learned running thousands of labs on thousands of people over a ten-year period. Importantly, I learned people have multiple complaints rooted in multiple causes. That is why we run multiple labs to investigate healing opportunities in the HIDDEN areas. We call this methodology Functional Diagnostic Nutrition® (FDN). That is the name of our company and the name of the course that we teach.

H-I-D-D-E-N stressors are found far upstream, and they often do not seem related to the symptoms that a person might have. So, the beauty of our system is that it is not symptom-based. Once we discover what's wrong or something that needs improvement, only then do we suggest a self-directed remedy a person can apply themselves, with good coaching of course. I started with the idea that *we* are responsible for our own health, and we need to take charge of our own healing. If we don't, others are happy to take charge for you.

One thing we learned in the last couple of years: If you don't take control of your health, others will. It would be good for them if you fall into their hands, but not good for you. We are in favor of people taking responsibility and overseeing their own health. The FDN system and methodology was developed with a self-care, empowerment, self-reliant mentality and has constantly evolved. It took 10 years to figure out the pattern listed above and prove how well it works. Now hundreds of FDN Practitioners and their clients know too.

Our Foundational Lab: The Stress and Hormone Panel

I started testing with hormones. At the turn of the century, most of the people coming into our clinic were middle-aged or older women, and hormones were important to them. They are important for men too, but women seem to care more about their health. At least, women pay more attention to their boo-boos than men.

I did thousands of hormone tests for our patients. Most were suffering with multiple complaints. Most women got a lot better; some got a little better. The major areas of their interest were perimenopause and post-menopause, bone density, libido, energy, and "hormone issues." I began by running a saliva test for circadian rhythm, catabolic/anabolic balance, and sex hormone levels, which we call the Stress and Hormone Panel. I ran my first salivary hormone test in the last century, and this stress lab has evolved nicely over the last couple of decades.

On one simple, inexpensive, at-home saliva test we look at several other markers along with the sex hormones because they are very interrelated. We measure cortisol and DHEA

(Dehydroepiandrosterone). These can tell us whether a patient is in a catabolic state or not and how seriously the body is breaking down.

Metabolism can be categorized into two main areas; catabolic activity, which is your body breaking down, and anabolic activity, which is your body building up. These activities should be in balance. The main catabolic hormone is cortisol, which breaks your body down. The main anabolic hormone we look at is DHEA, which counter-regulates cortisol and helps build you up.

We find a remarkably high correlation between feeling lousy or being full of "mystery complaints" and your body being in a catabolic state. In other words, when your cortisol level is too high in relation to your DHEA. This *catabolic dominance* is quite common and easy to see when you use the right lab work, and the self-directed remedy becomes obvious.

We also investigate the daily rhythm of the cortisol. In a "normal" rhythm, the cortisol is highest in the morning. It drops down at noon, drops down further in the afternoon, and goes even lower at nighttime. The balance between catabolic and anabolic is particularly important, but this look at the daily *circadian* rhythm is another key to understanding why people have health complaints. Evaluating the circadian rhythm requires measuring cortisol four times in a day, which is amazingly easy to do with a saliva test. You simply put your saliva in some little tubes when you wake up, again at lunch time, in the late afternoon, and once again before bedtime. Through this process, we get some useful information about a person. We learn why they are running out of energy or why they are not sleeping well and get many other insights. All these little insights can be capitalized on as they are used to guide a protocol.

Once you understand that you are in a catabolic state and your circadian rhythm is off; you can remedy all these things, mostly with lifestyle changes. That is the beauty of our work. We do not just medicate or treat the paper. We get the person to understand *why* they are in that condition; as well as what they can do to take charge of getting out of that condition and becoming a healthier and happier person.

The same simple saliva test, which has already given us a lot of information, can also tell us about the estrogen, progesterone, testosterone, and melatonin levels. The *sex* hormones: estrogen and progesterone, are often the main concern of women, although they also need to pay attention to testosterone levels. Not only do we uncover very low levels, but the levels are often found to be very much out of balance with each other. Through our self-directed method, we can all upgrade our hormones and our health. While you are not able to change your chronological age, you can feel much younger, healthier, and more vibrant when you function like a younger person.

Also From One Salivary Test: The Immune System and Secretory IGA

After 10 years of running thousands of labs and working with thousands of people, one of the principles I learned was that when someone has any kind of complaint, we cannot just say, "Here's your fix, take these pills." We need to look at the entire person if we are going to help them heal completely.

What I noticed in people with low hormones or with hormone imbalances, especially those in a stressed-out, catabolic vs. anabolic state, is that the next thing to become dysfunctional is the immune system. In another writing, I will explain the domino effect more thoroughly and how things can spiral downhill from there.

We all know people get sicker more often and do not recover as fast when they are stressed out. Thankfully, we were able to add another marker to our Stress and Hormone Panel to give us an idea of how things are going with the immune system. There is a salivary marker named Secretory IgA that lets us know how our immune system is doing.

Secretory Immunoglobulin A (Secretory IgA or SIgA) is the richest immunoglobulin (antibody) made in the body. It is the first line of defense against ingested pathogens and germs. SIgA is made just under the lining of the intestines and migrates through surface cells into the gut interior to become part of the mucous layer covering the lining of the intestines. That's a good thing. But SIgA can be suppressed by an elevated cortisol to DHEA ratio, or stress! And that's a bad thing. No wonder stressed out people are caught in an endless cycle of trial and error, frustrated, with nowhere to turn until now.

The immune system consists of many parts that work together to defend the body against invaders. It is generally accepted that the mucosal barriers throughout the body are critical and contain up to 80% of our immune system, especially the mucosal barrier of the gut, where SIgA reigns supreme.

You've heard here that people with chronic stress-related conditions due to multiple causes and multiple forms of stress are caught in a "downward spiral." I'm here to tell you that the more we explore this idea, the more we can observe a natural progression or pattern in the breakdown that is occurring. All with just a few simple lab tests that *anyone* can do.

We know the gut is an enormous part of the immune system and that SIgA plays a huge part. We know that with chronic stress, we often see depressed levels of SIgA and resultant weakened immunity. The next observation we make, and what appears to me as a natural progression in the breakdown of a person, is the breakdown in the composition of our gut flora or *microbiota*. From there, we see multiple pathogens move in or overpopulate the gut, eventually leading to gut permeability. The domino effect continues to break down the body. What comes next is another chapter for another book.

Last But Not Least: Melatonin

Our single saliva test can tell us we are out of catabolic/anabolic balance, how badly the circadian rhythm is disrupted, how much our sex hormones are out of balance, and as we have seen, how our immune defenses have been compromised.

Melatonin is also a key indicator of dysfunction. Using the same salivary stress and hormone panel, we get our melatonin level from the noontime sample when it should be at its lowest level. Elevated noontime melatonin is one more indicator of circadian rhythm issues and points the finger at gut dysfunction. It is also quite easy to correlate out-of-range melatonin levels, even low levels, with a variety of symptoms, including but not limited to sleep problems.

By now I hope you see why we run functional lab tests and why we say people caught in the downward spiral have multiple complaints due to multiple causes. For those who don't have a nagging health concern, and just want to increase vitality and vibrancy, or to just live longer, the same methodology applies.

Last words

I am a teacher, and my purpose is to put people back in control of their own health. It is difficult to find that in modern medicine because it is so focused on one thing: treating the symptoms. We need to look at ourselves as whole beings, including body, mind, spirit, and energy.

We must address all these functions and dysfunctions simultaneously through creating a proper epigenetic and lifestyle program. Through proper diet, rest, exercise, stress reduction, and supplementation, a better life can be achieved. FDN represents the ultimate lifestyle medicine program, and you get to practice it on yourself when you have the correct lab data to guide you. In this chapter, we looked at just one functional lab with multiple markers identifying multiple healing opportunities. I hope you will follow along as we explore other labs in chapters yet to come.

Reed Davis

CHAPTER 2: Find Your Triggers

By Pantea Kalhor, Publisher, Five Times Bestselling Author, FDN Practitioner, Certified Fertility and PTSD Coach

I had the privilege of spending a few days with my relatives who were mostly in their 60s and 70s. Each of them followed some traditional herbal remedies and lifestyle changes to manage their health issues. I was impressed by how a 70-year-old lady could manage her cancer and muscle pain to some extent, through taking regular workouts and losing some weight, but watching her eat sweets, white bread, and processed foods on a regular basis made me talk about what I learned in my FDN (Functional Diagnostic Nutrition) education and how I controlled my asthma and hormone imbalances by following the right diet and discovering the root causes through functional labs. Unfortunately, it is not easy to convince people to change habits they have been used to following for years. One day, when the 70-year-old lady worked with her hands, her arthritis pain locked her fingers, and she couldn't even hold a knife to peel an apple. I asked her if she knew her triggers and how she controlled her pain. She answered, "I don't take any pills or treatment for my pain. I live with it; it comes and goes." Despite trying to follow a healthy lifestyle, she still had some unhealthy habits and was really insistent on continuing what she believed. On the top of the wrong diet, her complex health issues were also being triggered due to losing her young daughter recently. We will dig into the relationship between trauma and overall health in the following pages.

The older we get, the more we become concerned about our health, because gradually our energy declines and our body gets tired of trying to adjust. We get tired of fighting and our body starts showing more imbalances and more symptoms; those inform us of deeper health issues which we may carry and ignore for years.

Our body has a magical self-healing power and tries to get to **homeostasis status or balance** (you can find more explanation in Chapter 3 about homeostasis). When we are younger, this power can still cover our pain and balance the body if we haven't carried any autoimmune disorders, serious infections, or genetic pain since birth. That ability may deceive us for some time. We may often hear people indicating that they are fine because their body always tries its best to stay in balance. The cycle continues until we misuse that power through our ignorance and delegate all responsibilities to our self-healing capacity and force it to balance the body. We are not aware of how we harm our health by continuing bad health habits and ignoring our pains and symptoms.

In this chapter, I aim to talk about different kind of triggers that act as blockers for our overall health and why we need to investigate root causes and healing opportunities rather than treating the lab results.

Emergency Versus Permanent Relief

I was rushed into the ER (Emergency Room) three times. Two times due to asthma attacks and once for a fatal miscarriage. What medicine did in all three cases was prevent my death or diminish my pain through immediate care and temporary remedies. These treatments are useful on the verge of life and death, but they will cause irreparable outcomes if they are repeated frequently. Let's say, if you don't treat your asthma and must rush into the ER now and then, you would be treated with steroids, drugs, and painkillers. The last time I went to the ER, the emergency doctor gave me a big warning and strongly emphasized following up with specialists after my release from the hospital. I knew I couldn't call the ambulance whenever I had an asthma attack, and my inhaler couldn't be effective all the time. I needed a remedy beyond the asthma inhalers.

Let's clarify the situation with this example. While driving, if one of your tires suddenly goes flat, you pull over and replace it with the spare tire. However, it may only help you drive enough to reach a mechanic to fix or change your tire. The spare tire may not be safe for the daily commute or a long trip. Painkillers and immediate fixes act like spare tires. They are safe enough to save you from death or an acute condition, but they can't heal you.

Painkillers and tranquilizers may create lots of trouble for you in the long run. ***Temporary relief can't offer permanent treatment.*** You need to build up your health foundation to fight against your health issues.

The reason you have a CBC (Completed Blood Count) test is to discover infection or pain by testing the white blood cell counts. The number of white blood cells increases to fight infection. Painkillers will mute white blood cells and stop them from growing. The body won't be able to generate antibodies, and our immune system starts weakening. I call it the gradual death of cells and body. When we consume painkillers in the long run, we are muting the warning signals and natural responses to our pain. The pain still exists; however, it remains hidden until we are triggered with the cause again. As I mentioned before, in case of emergency, that's the first thing to do, but in the long run we will be transformed to an addicted weak person who can't even tolerate a simple cold or flu.

Why are Common Lab Results Not Enough?

The conventional way that we all may choose is to visit our medical doctors for health complaints. Depending on your medical history, they may order some common lab tests such as CMP (Complete Metabolic Panel), a Lipid Panel, or a CBC. These tests are covered by insurance. They are inexpensive and accessible and aimed at determining your vitamin, mineral, or nutrient deficiencies or looking for infection, liver or bladder dysfunction, food and environmental sensitivities, digestive inflammation, chronic infection, and intestinal parasites. They are also aimed at supporting the diagnosis of a disease based on medical patterns and symptoms. It sounds great, right? But it's not that simple. When medical doctors find the specific pattern, two scenarios may happen.

1. You might be in a critical condition which needs immediate attention; they diagnose you with a disease, ask you to visit a hospital right away, or refer you to another specialist for more specific tests or treatment.

2. What if your tests show normal results? You would be sent off home with prescriptions for pills such as painkillers, vitamins, and supplements. In some cases, your medical doctor may only recommend that you reduce stress. On one hand, you would be happy that you didn't have a serious illness. On the other hand, you still have doubts and pains, and your problem has not been

solved yet! So, the question is **why, with all those normal results from laboratory tests, do you still not feel normal?** Are these pills, vitamins, and supplements enough to reduce your pain and offer a permanent solution to your health concern?

I respect Western medicine and the science that saves so many lives every day. I appreciate all the years of education and hard work that medical doctors have sacrificed to make this world a healthier place. However, digging into my health issues for fertility and asthma concerns made me investigate my own medical labs. I was going to find the answer to why, with all these tests and spending huge amounts of money on treatments, I couldn't get pregnant, or I had to rely on my inhalers to take a breath.

As a result of my journey, I would like to highlight a few facts here.

The **first fact** is that normal ranges in common labs are based on the average population, who are not completely healthy. So, the range is too broad to be able to pinpoint the problem. Let's have an example. **Uric acid** is one of the elements in a CMP. The normal range in the conventional medical laboratory is 3.5-7.2 (mg/dl); however, for the functional lab, the optimal range stands between 3.5-5.9 (mg/dl) for male and 3-5.5 (mg/dl) for female. So, if your uric acid has been measured as 6.1 (mg/dl), most probably you would be sent off home as a normal person. However, if you were measured by the functional optimal range, your uric acid level is not only abnormal but higher than the optimal range. That means your body has already started developing high uric acid symptoms. If not in the present, then in near future, your body would be on the edge of developing arthralgia, atherosclerosis, or renal insufficiency.

You may even have a leaky gut[1], or Mycotoxin (yeast)[2], heavy metal toxicity, inflammation, or liver dysfunction that will never get investigated at the right time.

Unfortunately, you will only be aware of your health issue when you have serious symptoms, and you are in a disease state.

So, in this scenario, since you have been told that you are normal, you will continue eating what you are not supposed to eat. Even if you try to take vitamins and eat organic and healthy foods, when your body has started developing a leaky gut, or renal or liver deficiency, how can taking vitamins help you when your body is not able to absorb them properly?

Second fact: usually people suffer from a combination of diseases, especially in the case of autoimmune disorders. Relying on a specific pattern for diagnosing a disease based on symptoms and the lab results may keep you from finding other healing opportunities in your body. We will discuss this more in detail later.

---

[1] Leaky Gut Syndrome: Symptoms, Diet, Tests & Treatment (clevelandclinic.org)
[2] Mycotoxins (who.int)

Third fact: you are the one who should be responsible for your own health in the first place. When I asked my doctor why he didn't go deeper in finding the hidden layers in my body, he said, "We can't examine your gut or liver for asthma. You only have a lung issue."

Becoming a healthy version of you needs work, dedication, and additional functional labs to test for hidden causes, which are not done in a usual conventional medical checkup.

Getting back to the uric acid example, do you think taking medication to lower the uric acid is enough? You may think a common way is to treat the paper, so the next time you visit your doctor, the results look better because your uric acid is lower. Are you happy now? How do you know if you have leaky gut, or renal or liver deficiency? What about heavy metal toxicity? Do these problems go away, and how can you investigate them?

You may have heard the same scenario for thyroid issues. Patients try to control their thyroid by treating the lab results. Thyroid may need another chapter to discuss, but I always use it as an example in my workshops and speaking engagements.

Just to summarize, thyroid issues could have originated from the hypothalamus, pituitary dysfunction, a binding and conversion issue (converting T4 to free T3) in the liver, cell dysfunction, or, believe it or not, gut disorder or dysbiosis[3]. Taking thyroid pills for hypothyroidism or hyperthyroidism only gives you a bit of relief and temporary aid. However, you may need to find the real root cause for your thyroid issue and not just treat the surface issue.

Functional labs have been tested on thousands of people for years and have proved that the optimal range is much narrower than what has been written on conventional laboratory papers. The fact is functional medicine is not going to treat any disease or balance the laboratory paper. We are looking for ways to find the hidden layers behind your discomfort in your whole body.

Connectivity in a Wider Spectrum

Based on what was discussed, holistic medicine firmly believes, not only all parts of the body are related to each other and function as a whole system, but our mind, body, and soul are also interrelated. If we are mentally and spiritually stressed or traumatized, the body stores the trauma at a cellular level, and that's the beginning of forming cancerous cells or chronic pain.

In a bigger spectrum, we, as humans, are related to each other. The environment and society affect our health. These recent years of Covid proved to us how one tiny virus, which could not even be

[3] Dysbiosis - an overview | ScienceDirect Topics

seen with our eyes, could create lots of damage. One diminutive virus made one person sick, and that one person threatened the whole world. Everyone guarded against others to be protected and safe. Countries were united to find the remedy because that was not only one tiny virus, but also a pandemic infection which needed global awareness and response.

If you wish to investigate your health issue, you may need to look at it in a broader spectrum and learn more about your environment.

Does your house have mold? What about your region or city? Are you living in a polluted area? The toxins are not only limited to physical toxins but include emotional toxins. Are you in direct contact with negative people? Do you live with financial difficulties? Do you hate your job or your life?

There are so many external factors which can create hidden layers for our health concerns and slow down our healing process.

The Power of Focused Energy

If you tend to stay in bed for long hours, you have low libido, and don’t have enough energy to go to work or perform your daily tasks, then you may need to discover your issue at a much deeper level.

Talking to my fertility clients, I try to point to energy as part of our discovery session. Many women suffer fatigue and energy shortages because they don't know how to manage this vital reserve. One of the biggest factors in losing energy for women without kids is too much focus on their career, spending long hours commuting to work, and on top of that, spending hours cooking, keeping the house clean, and doing other household duties.

I found the pattern for parents who suffer from secondary infertility issues, meaning they can't get or stay pregnant after having their first kid. I witnessed how raising their kids and managing their tantrums could increase their stress hormones and imbalance the whole body. They need to do more housework and keep their finances in balance. All that wastes the energy they need to get or stay pregnant and grow a healthy baby in their womb.

Mitochondria are membrane-bound cell organelles (mitochondrion, singular). They that generate most of our chemical energy needed to operate the cell's biochemical reactions. **They** act as units of energy in our body. We recharge these batteries by learning how to produce more energy and avoid wasting it. For more information about mitochondria, you can refer to the appendix.

We may have another interpretation for energy. As we discussed earlier, glucose is the fuel of your body. Some people try to compensate for their energy shortage by consuming sugar since they assume that's the initial source of energy in their body. Carbohydrates also transform into sugar, so excessive consumption of sugary products and carbohydrates not only doesn't boost your energy, but also makes you more exhausted since they will store in your body cells as fat and slow down your metabolism. They eventually imbalance your hormones and take the lead in exhausting you, mentally and physically.

I was analyzing test results for one of my clients, which showed some muscle atrophy. With the level of exhaustion she had, it was obvious her body was in a catabolic state, which showed as her body breaking down, along with hypothyroidism and other hormone imbalances. You can refer to Chapter 1 for more details about the catabolic/anabolic state.

In the functional medicine world, we change the adrenal fatigue term to metabolic chaos. Any imbalance in your body, no matter if it originates from glucose imbalance or dysfunction in the hypothalamus, pituitary gland, nervous or immune system, hormones, limbic system, liver, detoxification and binding, thyroid, or inflammation, may result extra stress and lead to exhaustion and fatigue [4].

---

[4] Is adrenal fatigue "real"? - Harvard Health

Healing needs focused energy. You can't initiate your healing process if you consume antidepressant pills or feel exhausted, sad, and negative. You also waste focused energy by distracting yourself with overthinking, a dark mind, or boring and repetitive tasks.

The healing starts from you. You need to stop wasting your energy and find more creative ways to avoid redundancies. It is essential to perpetuate your internal motivation to keep fighting, releasing, and reviving. I always recommend doing something creative that makes you happy. Remember, what you need is focused energy. When you stay away from distractions and are being innovative, your body starts secreting serotonin, dopamine, and oxytocin, or, in other words, happy hormones. That's the beginning of your healing journey.

When your body, mind, and spirit unite for healing, this centered energy helps you find ways to feel better. You need to collect all your forces to create a powerful stimulus.

It is necessary to be connected to your medical doctor, psychologist, or health care practitioner to get better results. If you start a treatment with doubt and distrust, or you don't have a good feeling about your therapy or your doctor, you are betraying yourself. If somebody else had a good result from a specific treatment, that doesn't mean you can benefit from the same treatment unless you believe in it. For example, I believe in acupuncture and functional medicine because they helped me have my baby, balance my hormones, and feel much happier and healthier. Research about the health care practitioner or the treatment. Listen to testimonials and find people who have already experienced the treatment.

Due to all the disappointing statistics, I overheard from my fertility doctor, I was not really connected to her or the IVF protocols she recommended. So, I chose an alternative way after two years of unsuccessful treatment. That doesn't mean IVF is not good for others. That means I deeply knew that there would be another solution for me. (If you would like to learn more about my fertility journey, you can go to my website: (http://panteakalhor.com) and order my book *Naturally Conceived* through Amazon.)

I recommended acupuncture to one of my friends. Since she didn't see any good results from other holistic medicine approaches for her mother's treatment, she didn't even bother to start any modalities like acupuncture for herself. She was not even open to hear or research about integrative medicine.

I mostly try to highlight the importance of holistic medicine and putting the necessary components together to build a meaningful health foundation. You may need to discover where disconnection takes place on your end. Take a piece of paper and write your answers. Is this between you and your lifestyle, your body, mind, and your spirit? Is this between you and your healthcare practitioner? Do you feel the chosen treatment may not be right for you? Do you have other external driving factors?

You may get lots of discouragement from your family, statistics, or other peripheral reasons. However, I saw evidence of how the power of centered energy helped a stage 4 cancer patient and a lady who suffered from multiple sclerosis recover from pain and get back to normal. So, you may need to meditate and find the courage to investigate your own health issues. You also need to take responsibility for generating the focused energy.

Let's Escape the Loop

As I stated in the previous section, everything in our body is related to other parts. If we try to treat the paper, we get involved in an infinite loop of trial and error, unless we can find a way to escape the loop. Okay, let's look at this pattern. When your sodium level increases, your potassium level decreases. The adrenaline hormone, aldosterone, helps regulate the sodium balance. High sodium causes **Adrenal Hyperfunction** [5]. Chloride (an electrolyte in the blood) maintains the body fluid balance and PH. Changes in chloride lead to changes in sodium and potassium level. High chloride is a sign of

[5] Adrenal Hyperfunction (Cushing Syndrome) Testing Algorithm | Choose the Right Test (arupconsult.com)

metabolic acidosis: the buildup of acid in the body due to kidney disease or kidney failure and chemical sciatica. Low chloride is a sign of low stomach acid and that causes H. pylori [6]. This list goes on and on. The imbalance in one mineral, vitamin, or electrolyte may create a lot of other imbalances in your body.

Another example would be glucose, which is the blood sugar in your body. Glucose is a fuel to the body's activities and its role is to support fat, protein, and carbohydrate metabolism.

Endorphin is the stress response hormone. They are released when your body in pain or stress. When we are in fight and flight mode, endorphin enhances the blood sugar and slows down digestion[7].

The pancreas halts its secretion of glucagon and releases insulin, a hormone that signals the body cells and the liver to take up glucose from the blood. On one hand, we need glucose to produce energy. On the other hand, the excess glucose will store in the body as fat and slow down our body metabolism.

You see how your body's organs, enzymes, hormones, and minerals cooperate to keep the body in balance. We can't separate one organ from another as they are functioning together as a whole.

---

[6] Helicobacter pylori (H. pylori) infection - Symptoms and causes - Mayo Clinic

[7] Endorphins: What They Are and How to Boost Them (clevelandclinic.org)

Cortisol: A Hidden Marker in Most Chronic Pain

At the age of 29, I had no sign of asthma, until I started taking open-water diving lessons for fun. (I have explained this trauma in the first book of "The Gap" series.) I was almost drowning when the instructor pulled out the oxygen mask. For a minute, I had forgotten to put my oxygen mask back on my face. I was scared to death about whether I could breathe again or not. When I survived, I promised myself I'd enjoy my life to the fullest and celebrate every second of it. However, since then, I started showing some signs of asthma. I thought I was released from trauma but that was deeper than I thought. I managed my breath with inhalers and referred to asthma and allergy experts. Unfortunately, none of them could help me get rid of the inhaler. I thought the only way was to use it forever. Even the allergy doctor never told me I might have inflammation or food allergies. He said I might be sensitive to flowers and seasons. Once I started learning about functional medicine, I asked my family doctor if he could test my cortisol level. He laughed and said, "We never order hormone tests for asthma."

While studying FDN, I ordered all five common FDN labs to test my body for cortisol and steroid hormones, melatonin, GI mapping[8], and the MWP (Metabolic Wellness Panel). I was in shock to see how low my cortisol level was. Even my melatonin and my steroid hormones like estrogen and progesterone were out of whack. During

[8] GI-MAP | GI Microbial Assay Plus | Diagnostic Solutions Laboratory

the pandemic, after the second dose of the Covid vaccine, my asthma attacked me again, and I had to restart my treatment to detox my body and boost my immune system.

What is usually missed are checking cortisol, the adrenaline profile and hormone panel, the GI map, and MWP. What has been blocked in asthma is not only respiratory tracts that may need inhalers to open. Asthma is mostly a reaction to inflammation, allergies, and toxins. Your hormone imbalance affects your asthma. Your gut and digestion issues may trigger asthma as well. We try to calm down and get away from fight-or-flight mode, and the inhaler only offers an immediate and temporary remedy. It adjusts the cortisol level without discovering why the level is imbalanced and what has caused the acute state.

I learned about my triggers and inflammation and why I should avoid certain foods and toxins, which could bring me allergies and inflammation. Knowing your body and discovering the root cause helps you find the missing piece of your health issue puzzle and build a stronger immune system.

One Common Mistake About Diet

Your diet is like a smoking habit. If you quit smoking for years and one day at a party with friends, you start smoking again, you can easily irritate your body against it. Since you have tried smoking again, you may repeat it at another party, or even another time when you are alone. You might say to yourself, "That's only one time to try." However, having broken your commitment, you will repeat this "one time" on more occasions.

It's the same with eating sugary and processed products like cakes, candy, and cookies. Avoiding your triggers should be part of your lifestyle. As soon as you have some replacement to enjoy eating, you can manage your temptation.

I was addicted to coffee and cakes, but since I quit drinking coffee, if I try it once, I can't sleep at night and my stomach hurts. I have the same reaction to sugary products. Not only do I not like or enjoy them anymore, but also, I have found other options which make my body happier and healthier. I don't need to add sugar to everything to enjoy the taste. I prefer to enjoy the real taste of what I eat.

How to Find Your Hidden Triggers

Finding the missing puzzle piece in your health mystery demands some discoveries about your triggers. Being tested by common labs may give you a rough estimation of what's going on in your body but if you are not tested based on the functional optimal range, you will miss the healing opportunity. Some medical and naturopath doctors who are aware of optimal ranges get a better result for their patients. They believe in holistic medicine since they have seen the results for their own health, their families, or their patients.

Following a diet plan without knowing your body and your triggers may endanger your health. So, what do we do next?

You can learn about functional labs to investigate your health issue and find healing opportunities. In the first chapter, with Reed Davis, we talked about it in more detail.

After examining your whole body, a FDN practitioner uses a DRESS (Diet, Rest, Stress reduction, Supplement) program to work with you to find healing opportunities. Note that this is not going to be an easy and fast recovery. FDN is not a substitute for other medical care and is not going to present a quick fix. Depending on your case, it may take more than three months to see the real result. That period varies in individuals and may take much longer, but the point is that more stable and permanent results need more dedication and commitment. Building a strong health foundation is not an easy and fast path; it takes time. It's exactly like when you try to build muscle. You can't build it in one day. You need a constant commitment to a regular workout, a healthy diet, enough rest, being relax and if needed getting right supplements.

Even if your health issues are the result of a big sudden emotional or physical injury, your chronic health issues have not been created in one day. They are the result of accumulated different untreated health issues in the long run.

It is Not Only One Health Issue

I often discover patients with one diagnosed chronic pain or autoimmune issue may have other undiscovered serious problems in their body. I talked to a woman who had a puffy face and recently was diagnosed with liver congestion. I asked her if she also had thyroid issues and her answer was yes. She started taking pills for hypothyroidism. Unfortunately, it is not easy to convince people to look for the root cause in their entire body as they can't believe thyroid issues may have roots in the gut or liver. In her case, she needed some liver detoxification at first.

As we explain in Chapter 4, Heather Gray, who is now a strong advocate about Lyme disease, not only struggled with Lyme, but also celiac and endometriosis. She will talk about how she reversed her autoimmune issues and feels much happier and healthier now.

Ignoring Your Health Issues in One Stage of Your Life Will Get Worse as You Get Older

So many couples try to conceive, but they don't believe that their fertility issues may be rooted in other physical, emotional, or spiritual issues. They only focus on sex hormones and common fertility treatments rather than their overall health. Then, they give up pursuing their fertility issue and finding the root cause. Later, they announce that they don't really need to have any baby.

When I visit these couples in their late 40's or early 50's, most of them are dealing with thyroid issues, exhaustion, early menopause, brain fog, and liver issues. ***Infertility was only an alert to warn them to look for other, deeper issues in their body.***

The Role of Trauma in Chronic Illness

In the "PTSD Self-Healing" show and *PTSD Compass* book, I talked about PTSD and transgenerational trauma.

Along with 15 other health care professionals, medical and naturopathy doctors, and health coaches, I have talked about trauma as one of the big causes of chronic disease, MS (Multiple Sclerosis), infertility, autoimmune disease, and so forth.

Having a healing mindset, facing, and recovering from your past trauma, and controlling your emotions can also expedite your healing process.

Some emotional pains can't go away easily, since we can't forget the death of a loved one, or we can't forgive the memory of an abusive relationship. No matter how hard we try to exercise or self-medicate with supplements and food based on our knowledge, we still need to investigate the hidden causes of our health issues carefully, confront our past traumas, and manage them. For more information, you can find the book here.

https://acechoiceidea.com/funnel/ptsd-compass/

You can also find some practical exercises to release yourself from trauma in Chapter 4 of this book.

DNA is Not Only Physical Genomes

As stated, an unknown pain in your body may be rooted in a trauma which not only happened in your life but in your ancestors' lives.

The pain has transferred to you through your soul and your DNA. There are so many case studies showing that our body is powerful enough to recover itself even if we have inherited autoimmune and chronic disease from our DNA, but sometimes it needs a little support. If your parents or your grandparents have diabetes, you still have the power to control this issue or deactivate your gene. You all, as a family, consume the same food and live in the same environment, which may contain mold or toxins. Besides, you and your family face the same emotional stress. All those will also be added to your family's health history. The reason we have different **metabolic types** (Metabolic typing is the science which categorizes people's diet based on their body needs) may also get back to a few factors, such as our DNA and our ancestors, our blood type, and our body constitution. Some cultures are originally vegetarian, some are not. Some are okay with corn; some are better off with beef. Chinese medicine also can determine your proper diet based on your blood type and your body constitution. So, if you are looking for general dietary suggestions without knowing your **metabolic type**, you may not benefit from your diet the way your body deserves.

Note that at this point we can't reverse genetic defects, blindness, or deaf ears, but we are not victims of autoimmune disorders, asthma, most chronic pain, or cancer just because one member of our family carries it. Even if we can't find the root cause, we can still avoid causes and find more healing opportunities in our body to have a lighter, happier, and healthier life. In Chapter 5, we will discuss DNA in broader areas.

How to Prevent Unnecessary Surgeries

Sometimes, I feel sorry for some of my clients who visit me for advice when they have done all the treatments they have known, and nothing worked for them. One of my clients was diagnosed with a combination of health concerns and had to close her Fallopian tubes. She was worried about whether IVF could help her get pregnant. Her big regret was not finding a holistic way to treat her other body issues before she was forced to do the surgery on her Fallopian tube.

My father suffered from back pain and thought he had to have surgery. However, he found a well-known chiropractor, and with some regular exercise and diet changes, he didn't need surgery.

Recently, I talked to another client. She had a collection of chronic problems, including thyroid, gut issues, and unexplained infertility. While listening to her health complaints, I also discovered that she had to remove her gallbladder a few years back.

If we ignore our body signs when they try to talk to us and only rely on our magical self-healing power in the hope that we get better soon, we may face damages which are not going to be compensated.

Sometimes I would love to scream and say, "Please look at your body as a whole system. Finding healing opportunities in your body may prevent unnecessary surgeries and help you before it's too late." In the first book of "The Gap" series, Dr. Jordanna Quinn, Physician, Regenerative, Anti-Aging, and Functional Medicine, Rehabilitation, Osteopath, and Medical Aesthetics has talked about this topic in more detail.

Last Words

My purpose in writing this book is to awaken the mentality that little tweaks in your lifestyle and analyzing your healing opportunities all over your body may really help you reverse your pain and get rid of the cycle of trial and error.

We are not the victims of permanent pain. If pain comes and goes, if we are always exhausted, or if we can't enjoy our food, then we need to do something about it. A normal life is a pain free, happy, and healthy life. If you thrive in a joyful and extraordinary life, you need to have a passion for change in your heart and strongly commit to changing your unhealthy habits.

Visualize your beautiful, pain free, and happy life in a 10- to 15-minute meditation every day and commit to take care of yourself. Healing can't be forced from outside; it starts within you.

CHAPTER 3: Treating Autoimmune Disease with Chinese Medicine

By Tsao-Lin Moy, Licensed Acupuncturist, Traditional Chinese Medicine Practitioner, and Herbalist

I have a private practice clinic located in Union Square in New York City where I practice Acupuncture, Chinese Medicine and Energy healing modalities. My focus for the past 20+ years is helping women find better and natural ways to get pregnant so that they don't have to undergo invasive or painful procedures just to have a baby.

With all conditions there is always one symptom that is present and that is pain, be it physical, emotional, or spiritual.

Pain conditions are the number one complaint for which people seek medical attention. Chronic pain presents as even more complex because the longer a person is suffering the emotions and the energy becomes blocked and hooked into traumas.

If it is not from a specific injury or trauma, then we look at patterns that can be tied to hormonal imbalances and autoimmune conditions.

With chronic pain, often present is systemic inflammation, hormone imbalances, as well as poor sleep, digestive problems and undiagnosed autoimmune conditions.

Many women post baby delivery suffer daily with various types of pain and discomfort. Symptoms of postpartum depression can reveal there is an underlying immune condition along with, anxiety, sleep and digestion issues, which are interrelated.

Pain is difficult for people to live with long term. They will go to great lengths to get relief, which is also why there is an opioid crisis in North America.

So many women today have inflammatory conditions such as subclinical thyroid conditions, and low-grade infections that often do not get picked up by common lab testing and can prevent women or couples from conceiving. Looking at the whole health history helps me address healing the whole body, because often times there is something residual that they didn't heal from.

What is Autoimmune Disease?

When your body's immune system attacks your own tissues and organs, we call it an autoimmune disease.

The aim of this chapter is to present the power of acupuncture and Chinese medicine in treating chronic pain and autoimmune disease. We specifically discuss some case studies associated with reactive arthritis, lupus, Lyme, and fibromyalgia.

Case Study: Reactive Arthritis

One of my male patients had been diagnosed with reactive arthritis. This is an autoimmune disease where the joints become inflamed and swollen. Reactive arthritis develops after an infection and one of its main triggers is food poisoning.

This patient ate food at a barbeque and then got sick; he felt like he had a stomach bug, but shortly after that, he developed body aches and pains all over like a flu, which was followed with extremely painful joints, swollen to the point that he could barely walk.

In cases like this, an allopathic approach gives the patients anti-inflammatory medicines, steroids, and long-term immune suppressants. Those medications suppress the symptoms of the inflammation, but the gut is what really needs to be addressed.

The food poisoning disrupts the gut microbiome; then that causes a cascade and disruption of the immune system. Gut health needs to be rebalanced because it is intrinsic to immune support and resetting the nervous system. More stress emotionally and physically causes more inflammation, and it becomes a vicious cycle, which is often the case with autoimmune conditions.

We look for what triggers the condition, and that is a clue to what could be the root cause, and where to address healing. Sometimes using medication, itself causes a lot of inflammation, especially for women who are on birth control for years. They may end up taking a lot of antidepressants. This is because side effects of hormonal birth control are depression and low libido.

Even things we believe are healthy, like using supplements, need to be taken with caution; consuming many supplements at the same time can contribute to inflammation and trigger reactions.

The beauty of acupuncture and Chinese medicine is that we look at the "whole body" and do not treat just the symptoms. We start by looking at their whole health history. Oftentimes there are underlying conditions that get triggered. They may be from some chronic issues which patients have had for a long time.

The Chinese classics say that the deadliest illnesses have the smallest symptoms, so they go unnoticed until it is too late.

Western medicine looks more for a cause and effect versus something happening over time.

Diagnosing a disease is taking a group of symptoms, chunking them together, and labelling them. Chinese medicine will look at many diseases and the treatment principle will be the same because the underlying disease process is the same; it is a matter of recognizing the patterns. The more complex a "disease," the simpler the treatment principle.

When the accurate pattern is identified through TCM (Traditional Chinese Medicine) principles, we can find a root cause and treat that, even when it looks counter to the symptoms. Then we witness the person healing.

After each acupuncture session, they can feel the difference.

Let's have an example of one of those autoimmune diseases which is not easily diagnosed.

Fibromyalgia

Fibromyalgia is an autoimmune disease. Until recently, it was almost impossible to diagnose this autoimmune condition. The patients may have pain all over the body. It can mimic inflammatory conditions such as rheumatoid arthritis, lupus, and Lyme.

Fibromyalgia can also be accompanied by mental fogginess and sleep disturbance, psychological distress, depression, and irritable bowel syndrome. Recently, there have been much clearer ways to diagnose fibromyalgia, usually by excluding other illnesses that have more definitive test confirmations.

Fibromyalgia is the result of an inflammation of the connective tissue as well as the muscle tissue.

Studies show that psychological stress plays a role in pain and is linked with fibromyalgia and rheumatoid arthritis.

Treating Fibromyalgia Holistically Without Painkillers

Cultivating a balanced lifestyle and managing stress and stress hormones can help prevent and mitigate pain flare-ups. Since the pain might be felt all over the body, acupuncture and Chinese medicine can make a big contribution in treating fibromyalgia. Acupuncture and point needles can:

- Help reset the nervous system. As a result, it releases endorphins or "feel good" chemicals.

- It improves fluid circulation and lymph flow so that inflammation can be reduced.

- Enhances sleep quality.

- Eases pain.

- Alleviates stress.

- Supports the immune system.

Depending on whether pain is related to fibro and connective tissue or associated with muscles, Chinese medicine can discover the right channel to work with to relieve the pain.

Case Study: Lyme and Fibromyalgia:

Lyme disease is one of the most common causes of autoimmune disease. Lyme is contracted from a tick infected with the bacterium *Borrelia burgdorferi* and rarely, *Borrelia mayonii*. It is transmitted to humans through the bite of infected blacklegged ticks. In most cases, if caught very early, it can be treated with a few weeks of antibiotics.

However, sometimes there is no rash on the skin where the bite occurs, and unfortunately, it can't be caught early. It stays dormant for years and creates lots of problems in the body, such as fever, headache, fatigue, and a characteristic skin rash called erythema migraines. If left untreated, infection can spread to joints, the heart, and the nervous system. Lyme disease is diagnosed based on symptoms, physical findings (e.g., rash), and the possibility of exposure to infected ticks.

In the case of a tick bite and suspected Lyme, I fully support taking antibiotics immediately to get ahead of the spirochete life cycle.

Laboratory testing is helpful if used correctly and performed with validated methods, but by the time the test result comes back, a few

[9] Lyme Disease | Lyme Disease | CDC

weeks may have passed, and you might miss the window of early treatment[9].

I had a patient who has suffered from pain conditions for years. She was given a diagnosis of fibromyalgia and had undergone test after test, and even Lyme came up negative. The doctors were baffled and continued to treat her symptoms. As with all autoimmune conditions, stress makes inflammation worse, causing flare-ups.

This condition can come from poor diet, hormonal imbalances, not enough sleep, or an emotional stressor. Stress hormones like adrenaline and cortisol also feed the Lyme spirochete life cycle.

Lyme can also affect the endocrine system, and as female hormones naturally fluctuate, this becomes another set of symptoms to chase down and try to control.

With so many autoimmune conditions, it is a constant cycle of chasing and treating symptoms that just don't work, and in fact, create more havoc in the nervous system.

This is because the body becomes a battleground of fighting an elusive enemy and the result is pollution and destruction of the natural ecosystem.

How Did My Patient Discover That Lyme Disease Was the Culprit?

A sinus infection caused her to take antibiotics. During that time, she was retested, and the Lyme showed up!

She was undergoing a lot of medication to get rid of the spirochete[10]

which also created more stress on her system.

To withstand the antibiotic treatment cycles, she needed to strengthen her body and immune system.

The Treatment

As the first step, we needed to relax the nervous system because stress made everything worse. We also needed to create a stronger connection between mind and body to speed up healing. So, I recommended:

- Meditation: to relieve the stress.

---

[10] spirochete | Definition, Examples, Diseases, & Facts | Britannica

• Body movement: to help fluid circulation in the body, release endorphins, control emotions from the muscles, and get more connected with the body.

• Enough sleep to give time to the body to digest, detoxify, relax, produce, regenerate, and balance the hormones.

As the second step in treating her discomfort, I helped her body purge the inflammation and detoxify her body. In Chinese medicine as well as Western medicine, the liver is the organ that helps to detoxify the body and process metabolic waste, as well as clean the blood and regulate immune functions. The strategy is to support liver function.

Food plays a very important role in clearing inflammation as well.

I also recommend drinking tea.

Dandelion flower tea is beneficial for Sore throat and mastitis. It is also good for "heat" conditions such as bladder infections and inflammation. In Chinese herbal medicine, it is called *Pu Gong Ying* and is used in formulas for breast tenderness and mastitis with breastfeeding and detoxing the liver.

Studies [11] show that dandelion also helps with liver function and has anti-diabetic effects, which helps with blood sugar regulation.

---

[11] The Physiological Effects of Dandelion (Taraxacum Officinale) in Type 2

Third step focused on diet: removing inflammatory foods, like sugar, dairy products, artificial sweeteners, sodas, and processed foods. Eating whole, simple, organic foods and mainly plant based. This helps to reduce additional stress on the digestive system. Here are some guidelines.

1. Focusing on a plant-based diet where you have at least five varieties of vegetables and fruits.
2. Preparing your own food means you are conscious of and know about its origins.
3. Eating whole foods in season that are nutrient dense is working with the natural cycle of life.
4. No alcohol.

The US is the unhealthiest country globally. This is due to high obesity, diabetes, and heart disease. The Standard American Diet (SAD) is full of processed foods that are animal based, meats and dairy, as well as sugar. Processed foods, even those that purport to be healthy, are far from their original form and lose their nutritional value. The strategy is to make it as easy as possible for your body to synthesize and absorb nutrients that support health.

Diabetes - PMC (nih.gov)

There are certain foods that are considered superfoods that aid in immune support and neurological function such as mushrooms: Shitake, Reishi, Maitake, Lion's mane, and Cordyceps.

Choose foods that promote repair and antiaging and rejuvenation, such as mushrooms, grape seed extract[12], and Chinese Celery[13].

Word of caution: Since fibromyalgia is followed by fatigue, I try not to make the patient more exhausted by changing too much all at once. I look at their overall health condition and go through their health chart, which I create for each patient. Each person is different, and I may recommend different customized treatments based on the person's needs. The more exhausted they are, the less I use needles, and I recommend fewer herbs and supplements.

Many fibromyalgia patients experience depression, and pain is often treated with in tandem with anti-depressant drugs, which again cause the body more exhausted.

When guiding the body to heal we want to give simple messages and not overwhelm the body.

---

12 Grape Seed Extract - an overview | ScienceDirect Topics

13 A Review of the Antioxidant Activity of Celery (Apium graveolens L) - PMC (nih.gov)

Why are Women Prone to Fibromyalgia?

In the Western perspective, there are markers in the blood that may indicate autoimmune disease[14].

Chinese medicine knows that psychological stress plays a huge role in pain, which is linked to fibromyalgia and other conditions like rheumatoid arthritis and hormonal fluctuations. That may explain why women are twice as prone to fibromyalgia. Due to menstruation, menopause, or pregnancy, women suffer from more hormonal fluctuation. Chronic stress can diminish the immune system's ability to respond to and fight against diseases over time [15].

Are You A Type A Personality?

A "Type A" personality person is more prone to autoimmune conditions because they use stress and adrenaline to push their version of success on themselves.

Perfectionism and pushing to "the limit" are very Yang energy. Not allowing themselves to rest, restore, and rejuvenate is yin. They often suffer from adrenal exhaustion, crash, and ultimately, burnout.

---

14 https://www.verywellhealth.com/autoimmune-blood-test-5112938.
15 Why Women Are More Prone to Fibromyalgia: CHOICE Pain & Rehabilitation Center: Physical Medicine, Rehabilitation, and Pain Management

What these patients have in common with autoimmune disorder sufferers is that they are not connected to their body. They ignore when they are tired and instead will force themselves to work out, go without sleep, deprive themselves of regular meals, and then expect high performance.

There is an internal critic or task master that does not let them rest. *Striving for excellence is in our nature; however, working to exhaustion is a losing battle.*

Often this personality trait will have difficulty relaxing. They are anxious about the future and can become irritable. They experience angry outbursts and lose control of their emotions. When this happens, they tend to try to control more things and even people around them. A coping mechanism is focusing on "fixing" and perfectionism, as well as ritualistic behavior and obsessive cleaning. If you recognize some of these patterns in yourself, it is helpful to learn ways to develop a strong mind-body connection and self-care management. We are mindful of over-committing and multitasking[16].

[16] Personality and Fibromyalgia Syndrome - PMC (nih.gov)

Gluten Intolerance and Celiac Disease

Gluten intolerance[17] has become more and more common, affecting up to 6% of the US population. It is referred to as non-celiac gluten sensitivity (NCGS). With the increase of eating wheat and starch in the diet along with antibiotics in the food system, food sensitivities and allergies are on the rise. This translates to constant low-grade inflammation that the immune system registers as an attack.

Celiac disease (CD) is an autoimmune disorder that is estimated to affect one percent of the population. There are genetic factors that predispose certain people to developing this serious autoimmune condition.

The absorptive surface of the small intestine is severely damaged by the immune system's response to gluten. Gluten is a group of proteins present in wheat, rye, and barley.

Gluten sensitivity affects nutrition absorption, such as protein, fat, carbohydrates, vitamins, and minerals[18].

Even if fibromyalgia patients are not diagnosed with celiac disease, this study shows a great improvement in patients' conditions after choosing a gluten-free diet[19].

---

[17] Gluten Intolerance: Symptoms, Test, Non-Celiac Gluten Sensitivity (clevelandclinic.org)

[18] Celiac Disease - What is it? - Canadian Celiac Association

Case Study: Lupus

Lupus is another autoimmune disease which can mimic other autoimmune ailments. Inflammation caused by lupus can affect your joints, skin, kidneys, blood cells, brain, heart, and lungs. Infections, certain drugs, or even sunlight can be some of the causes of lupus flareups.

The signs and symptoms of lupus that you experience will depend on which body systems are affected by the disease. The most common signs and symptoms include fatigue, fever, joint pain, stiffness and swelling, shortness of breath, chest pain, dry eyes, headaches, confusion, and memory loss[20].

One of my patients had been diagnosed with lupus. Her body was inflamed and swollen, what I describe as squishy, and her face was puffy. Patients with Lupus often feel "unwell" and sluggish. In Chinese medicine this is called Damp Bi syndrome. Swelling and fluid is known as dampness and the inflammation as toxic water. The strategy is to remove the dampness and toxic water that causes the heaviness and sluggishness that continues to damage the body function.

---

[19] Fibromyalgia and non-celiac gluten sensitivity: a description with remission of fibromyalgia: https://www.ncbi.nlm.nih.gov/pmc/articles/PMC4209093/

[20] Lupus - Symptoms and causes - Mayo Clinic

(There is much more that is addressed on an individual basis which I won't get into for this case.)

There is an important exercise that I teach all my patients: how to stimulate their lymphatic system to move inflammation out of the body. It is a lymphatic drainage practice; a lymphatic reset with nine steps that I have adapted, including Tai Qi and Qi Gong practices. This supports moving the inflammation out of their system. They should do it one or two times a day, making it part of a morning practice.

My Nine-Step Lymph Reset

This self-massage, first thing in the morning, will quickly help detox the body by activating the lymphatic system. This sequence incorporates "pai da" or body tapping.

Technique: Massaging in circular motion, using the fingers like a claw, then patting/slapping the area like you would pat someone on their back.

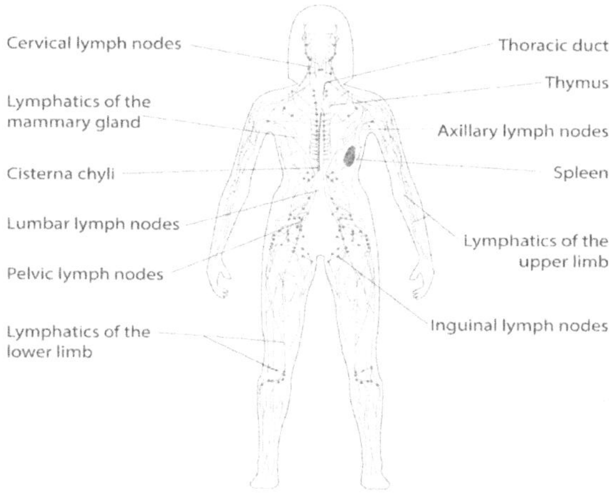

Figure 1: Lymphatic System

Sequence:

1. Above and below the clavicle in line with the nipple. Massage up and down and in a circular motion. Then pat the area like you are patting someone on the back.
2. At the angle of the jaw just below the ear on the SCM (synonym musculus sternocleidomastoid EUs), massaging circles from the top going down, then tap with fingertips from top to bottom.
3. (Three fingers) In front of the ears and (two fingers) behind the ears. Massage up and down and in small circles. Then gently tap the cheeks and neck down to the clavicle.
4. Armpit/axillary, grab the pectoralis muscle so that the fingertips are in the armpit, knead, massage it, and tug. Pat/slap the armpit.
5. Middle of the chest, massaging the front of the sternum as if there were frills on a shirt. Pound the chest like a chimp.
6. Below the ribcage, the entire belly area, big massage like a washing machine, moving from the sides toward the belly button, lower belly and upper stomach move toward the belly button. Jiggle and massage, then pat and slap the belly.
7. With hands in a loose fist, massage the lower back in circles and up and down, then pound the back like a drum.
8. Groin crease, crossing the inner crease with vigorous massage, then cupped patting/slapping.

9. Behind the knees: massage moving the skin, then slapping the back of the knees. Gentle jiggles, jump and shake your body.

Diet is also an important factor to reduce inflammation. Avoiding certain foods that are inflammatory, artificial sweeteners, and do not drink soda. We call it detoxification.

After the first treatment with acupuncture, my patient shared that she felt much lighter. The next day, after doing the lymph drainage reset, she reported that it felt like she was peeing out the fluid.

When patients feel relief in their treatment, they experience success and are motivated to pursue the process.

I believe we need to educate our patients on how they can take care of themselves, so that they can fully participate in their healing process. We are not with them when they are tempted to reach for potato chips or processed foods, that is the moment for them to make the healthier choice for themselves.

Some steps are simple and make sense for helping our overall health. For example, substitute drinking cow's milk with a plant-based alternative. Many people do not digest and metabolize dairy products. In addition, they are not a great source of calcium or vitamin D, regardless of what the dairy industry advertises.

Prepare and cook more of your own meals by choosing unprocessed and organic foods, exercise with activities that are fun and that you can do with other people and your children. Make sleep a priority.

This is about consciousness with self-care and cultivating habits that build health and resilience and ultimately your health span.

How Acupuncture and Chinese Medicine Support Homeostasis/ Body Balance?

Acupuncture stimulates the neuropeptides[21] that reduce inflammation and balance the nervous system. It is a non-pharmaceutical treatment, and it doesn't interfere with medication.

- Stimulating acupuncture points helps bring the body back into balance (the Yin and Yang within the body). The Western understanding would be homeostasis. Yin and Yang balance in Chinese medicine is not static, it is the state of dynamic balance.
- **Homeostasis is the state of balance that the** body's self-regulating mechanism moves toward.

[21] Frontiers | Neuropeptide and Small Transmitter Coexistence: Fundamental Studies and Relevance to Mental Illness (frontiersin.org)

- Think of homeostasis like a thermostat that regulates the temperature to be within an ideal range, no matter what fluctuations there are in the weather.
- When the body experiences illness, this is a symptom from the body struggling to attain homeostasis. In the case of autoimmune conditions, there is a constant battle with an invisible enemy, and it causes a dysregulation of the body's balancing system.
- Strong mind body connection. Being able to feel the energy move in your body and what it is like to really relax is experiencing a different way of being. The more connected and conscious you are to your body, the easier it is to be intuitive and make the best choices for yourself. If you are tired then don't push yourself, modify what you are doing and assess what could be contributing to the fatigue. If you eat certain foods and feel sick, then don't eat them.

Last Words: Awakening Natural Healing Abilities with Acupuncture

- *"The healer you seek is already inside you!"*
- Each person is born with natural inner healing abilities. The principles and practice of acupuncture and Chinese medicine understand how the body works and how to heal with balancing of Yin and Yang energy. **Yin and Yang balance**

addresses all aspects of the person: energetic, physical, emotional, and spiritual levels.

- **Pain** is a message to pay attention: something may be going on or there may be an imbalance inside your body. This is like the flashing light on a car that says, "Check engine." It is an opportunity to take care of something small so that it does not later become a big problem.
- I've heard so many times in my office, "I wish I knew this before, so I could have done something about it." Right now, is your future "before." Imagine yourself 10 years from now…what would you have liked to tell the younger version of yourself?
- Many autoimmune conditions are often rooted in past traumas, which may come to the surface years later in the form of pain or disease. They often have "mysterious" symptoms that come and go, like hide and seek.
- The brain can't differentiate between psychological and physical trauma. Events in your past may have created shock/trauma to your system, and this floods the body with stress hormones, registering in your cells as pain.
- Major life changes, both joyful and painful, can be stressors in our psyche. Stressful events such as death of loved ones, physical injury, or serious illness such as cancer, childhood trauma, job loss, abusive relationships, separation, or divorce

can put us in "survival" mode. What no one really talks about or addresses, is when women experience infertility. The psychological trauma of undergoing painful and invasive procedures to have a baby affect all aspects of a woman's life and relationships. Burying those events, so we can function, does not necessarily mean that we have processed them or fully healed from them.

- If you are in the throes of pain or autoimmune conditions, it is important that you don't give up hope of healing and feeling better. There are always things you can do on your own and by taking the action of reading this book you are moving towards health.
- A warning: If a medical practitioner tells you that you don't have a choice or that you will have to be on medication the rest of your life, you must believe that it is NOT the only truth. What they share is their own limiting belief of what is possible in health and healing. They are trained to look for how someone's illness will fit into a diagnosis and pharmaceutical model.
- You have the power to balance, heal, and regenerate yourself.

CHAPTER 4: Hidden Causes of Autoimmunity

By Heather Gray, FDN Practitioner

Heather Gray here, a.k.a. Lyme Boss. I was bitten by a tick when I was 13. (Ticks are parasites that feed on warm-blooded hosts by biting them. A tick bite can infect humans and animals with bacteria, viruses, and protozoans (organisms made up of one cell) that can cause diseases[22].

I started to develop symptoms when I was 15 and then ended up in the psych ward for the first time due to a suicide attempt. As I got older, I was in the psych ward another time for a suicide attempt. Sadly, both of those times all they ever wanted to do was throw prescriptions at me, pat me on the head, and send me out the door. Nobody was looking deeper into why I was not functioning properly. I also had gut issues. I was bloated and gassy, had bad skin and horrible periods. It wasn't until decades later, when I was 34 years old, that I finally got diagnosed with Lyme disease. I had it for over 28 years. As a result of a crazy chronic widespread pain, I

[22] Tick Bites: Causes, Symptoms, Treatment & Prevention (clevelandclinic.org)

visited roughly 10 to 20 different practitioners in a span of 10 years looking for answers.

All of them put me on different prescriptions. However, none of them talked to me about diet, lifestyle, stress level, mindset, and sleep. I didn't hear about any of that until I heard the founder of FDN (Functional Diagnostic Nutrition), Reed Davis, on a podcast talking about how we need to balance our hormones; why it is necessary to make sure our detox pathways are open; why we need to heal our gut; why it is necessary to remove hidden stressors in order for our body to take over and heal itself. I knew this was the course I needed to take and also the missing piece to my health puzzle. I had to change my direction; so, I studied the course and applied it to myself first. FDN completely changed my life. I lost around 80 pounds; I got out of chronic pain; I was no longer depressed and anxious; and I had the energy to enjoy spending time with my kid and my husband after a day's worth of work. I have reversed two out of three of my autoimmune diseases. What a blessing this is. I have stable moods; I'm not as reactive, snarky, and angry all the time. I could be like the Hulk and was set off easily. Can you relate?

FDN gave me my life back, and that's why I do what I do. That's why I got into this line of work: So that I could help bring others on their health journey and show them how they can be the boss of their own health journey.

The Combination of Pain I Suffered

I used to tell people on a scale of one to 10 (ten being horrible), I was living with a level six or seven pain on a regular basis. I remember once, a massage therapist asked me, "What kind of painkillers do you take?"

"Painkillers? Why would I take painkillers?"

"You just feel like you're in excruciating pain. Your muscles are rock hard."

I said: "I am. It just kind of made me a reactive and not a very nice person to be around. However, I would not take the prescription medications for that because I know how addictive they can be."

Lyme pain is weird because it tends to migrate and that's why it's so hard to pin down for a lot of folks; one day my right shoulder was painful; then, the other day it was my left knee. And some days it was like flu achiness everywhere.

I also had Hashimoto's, celiac and endometriosis, mold toxicity, and issues with heavy metals on top of Lyme disease and its co-infections.

I believe the reason I had this collection of pain was that I used to have a traditional Standard American Diet, including sugar and processed foods, known as the SAD diet; I also had early childhood trauma and a genetic predisposition for celiac. My lifestyle wasn't the greatest either. I was staying up too late. Stressed out to the max, wasn't drinking enough water, was constipated, and worked in an environment with lots of toxins. Since then, I have reversed two out of the three autoimmune diseases in me, endometriosis and Hashimoto's.

My Hashimoto's Symptoms and Reversal

When I had Hashimoto's, I was losing my hair in big chunks. It was really freaking me out. My feet and my hands were always cold, and I was exhausted. No gas in the tank. As I started balancing my body with what I learned in FDN, my hair was finally coming back; I had energy, and my extremities no longer felt like ice cubes.

Endometriosis Signs and Reversal

I had heavy and painful periods for decades. I thought my uterus was trying to kill me. I did have a partial hysterectomy done a few years back. If I knew what I know now, I would have been able to prevent that, but at the time I was not walking the walk I do now. Three decades' worth of getting my butt kicked every month, I was kind of over it. And again, I wasn't ready to live the clean lifestyle I do now. It is possible to reverse it, despite what your doctor may have told you. If you would like to learn more about endometriosis, you can check the following Web link. (https://www.hopkinsmedicine.org/health/conditions-and-diseases/endometriosis)

My Celiac Journey

I did not know that it was not normal to eat a bottle's worth of Tums (a famous medication for relieving stomach aches and heartburn) in two weeks. I also didn't know that it wasn't normal to carry Gas X (a popular over-the-counter medicine to help with gas and bloating) with you everywhere you go. I had a package of Gas X in my purse, in my locker at school, and in my car because the discomfort was horrible. After eating anything, it seemed like I would just bloat up like a balloon. I used to laugh and say that I was like Violet on *Willy Wonka and The Chocolate Factory* (an American movie back in 1971). I was waiting for Oompa Loompas to jump out, start singing a song, and roll me away to squeeze all that air out of me. It was being celiac and not knowing I was celiac that caused all that pain and embarrassment.

Looking back now, I realize I was basically born constipated. I was sitting on the potty at only four years old. I remember my feet falling asleep from sitting on the potty for so long. At the time, the doctors weren't trying to figure out what was wrong with this four-year-old and why she was constipated. They were just giving me these thick nasty oils to "soften my stool" and get me going. Between the Lyme and the celiac, I always had gut issues. There were times when I literally felt like I wasn't digesting anything; everything hurt, and everything caused inflammation. I was a hot mess and because of this, I also developed a weird relationship with food. In time I realized that the stuff that I was eating was not food. If you do not recognize an ingredient, neither does your body. Removing grains and other foods that cross-react with grains like dairy and corn was absolutely pivotal.

If I accidentally get cross-contamination somewhere, it affects my brain and other parts of my body for a week or two afterward; so, I don't even mess around with that anymore.

My son has celiac as well. He was diagnosed at the age of two. It is so bizarre that it took me another 10 years after his diagnosis before I figured out that I had it too, because there is a huge genetic component to it, but for some reason, I didn't connect the dots at the time.

Can You Conquer Your Genes?

Autoimmune issues can have a genetic component to them. And there is a relationship between epigenetics and how our DNA is affected (epigenetics is how our lifestyle and our environment affect our DNA expression). I absolutely do not believe that just because it's in your genes, it's final. There is an expression out there that *genes are the gun, and lifestyle is the bullets.* If you are leading this inflammatory and stressed-out lifestyle, the chances of you expressing those funky genes become much higher.

Wheat causes inflammation in almost everybody regardless of whether you have celiac or not. Every single person I have tested who has chronic health issues, depression, and anxiety also had issues with wheat and gluten as well. It is a toxic, processed food, dripping in pesticides, glyphosate, and other toxic chemicals.

Case Study: Reversing Lyme for One of My Clients

Recently I was working with a client who suffered from Lyme for over 25 years. I will call her Laura. Most of us with Lyme, especially when we carry it for decades, don't just suffer from Lyme disease. We suffer from co-infections, leaky gut, another autoimmune disease, heavy metal toxicity, and parasites. She gave me one of the best testimonials I have ever had so far. Laura said that she wished she had met me 16 years ago because what she had been able to do in the short four months since we started working together had gotten her better results than anybody else she's worked with.

Just from looking at the other hidden stressors in the body and building a healthy foundation. It is amazing what the body is capable of.

The part that distresses me the most is that in the Lyme community everybody is so focused on treatment, but nobody talks about the lifestyle. If you don't set up that healthy foundation, you are setting yourself up to relapse. I have done it myself. There's an awesome documentary called *A Monster Inside Me.* A lady talks about how she overcame Lyme with herbals; then she went back to her typical way of eating and stress levels and she relapsed. What I like to do with people, more than anything else, is to focus on getting the foundations.

I want to get them rock solid because whether it's Lyme, cancer, diabetes, or any other disease, setting up these foundations will help you improve dang near every single condition out there! Do not pass go, do not collect $200. You will go straight to bad health jail if you do not build a healthy foundation.

FDN focuses on the DRESS success model. That's the combination of Diet, Rest, Exercise, Stress reduction, and Supplementation. Supplements come at the end because you can't supplement your way out of a bad diet. Diet is the key; so, removing inflammatory foods that impact your blood sugar negatively is the first thing you need to do.

I am always surprised when I start working with someone who is on multiple prescriptions and I ask them, "What did your doctor say about lifestyle and diet?"

They look at me like I am crazy, "What do you mean, what did my doctor say about diet?"

I say, "Didn't they ask you about how you're eating or what your stress level was like?"

"No. They just met with me for 10 minutes and wrote me a prescription. Then they sent me out the door."

How do you help somebody heal when you just keep throwing band-aids at symptoms? Functional practitioners such as I dig a little deeper, take a little more time with folks, guide them, and really teach them how to become the "Boss" of their own health journey.

Rest or sleep is as important as dieting. What time do you go to bed at night? Are you on your mobile devices right before you go to bed? Do you have a hard time winding down? Are you sleeping with your cell phone next to your head? This is not healthy, by the way.

Healing requires deep, restful sleep because that's when our body starts repairing and healing. So many people who are chronically sick may skip this huge piece of the healing process; it is inexpensive – free! - by the way. Once you get that dialed, it's going to be one of your best tools to help your body recover and heal. I used to say silly things when I was younger, like, "I can sleep when I am dead." Sadly, not sleeping enough was going to bring me closer to death than I realized.

Another piece in my health puzzle was trauma work: somatic experiencing techniques and breath work. These exercises were necessary to move stored trauma out of my nervous system. Without it, your body is constantly in fight-or-flight mode like a tiger is always chasing you. Your energy isn't going toward healing when you're running away from a tiger; it is going to your extremities; it's going to your muscles, and it's taking the energy away from hormones and digestion. At the end of the day, it's taking the energy away from healing.

Your body is not thinking about having sex, or digesting food, or healing, for that matter, when you are under stress. It is thinking about getting away from that tiger. Maybe the tiger is your spouse, your stressful job, your kids, or the chronic disease that you might have in your body. Trauma and stress come in many forms, and it is imperative that you get that stress level under control. You need to reset your nervous system to truly heal.

Self-care is The Building Blocks of Your Health

I always emphasize how important self-care is and love teaching it. I am like a detox queen. I love castor oil packs, coffee enema, infrared sauna blanket, skin brushing, sunbathing, Epsom salt baths, intermittent fasting, and meditation.

1. Castor Oil Pack

I love my castor oil pack. My favorite regimen is to wear my castor oil pack on Thursday nights; they make these cool ones that you can wear overnight. It helps the liver detox and lowers inflammation. It helps regulate bowel movements, balance hormones, and improve sleep.

2. Coffee Enema

Then Friday morning, after wearing my castor oil pack, I do a coffee enema. The special kind of coffee helps the liver detox. "The primary function of a coffee enema is **to remove toxins and waste from the body**.

Caffeine increases enzymatic activity in the intestine. It helps flush out toxins, thereby giving your body the nutrients to heal. It also lowers inflammation, restores bowel function, and increases energy levels.[23]"

3. Infrared Sauna Blanket

An infrared sauna blanket is another favorite detox I regularly do. First, I do some skin brushing and then get into the sauna blanket. It is just such a powerhouse of detoxification. I like to do skin brushing before an Epsom salt bath as well. Sweating is one of my favorites. It helps the body detox, especially when you have mold issues and poor genetics that do not allow you to detox properly, as I do.

---

23 https://colon90210.com/blog/coffee-enemas-are-they-worth-it

4. My Special Way of Meditation

Meditation is another beneficial self-care method. I use it and recommend it to my clients as well; however, I do it a bit differently from other regular meditation techniques.

I record my voice saying positive words; then I listen to the recording every day. Most people with chronic illnesses have some drama component to it which ties into some negative self-talk. My whole life, I was no stranger to beating the snot out of myself; I was my own worst enemy most of the time. So, I knew if I wanted something different, I needed to learn some new tools and that was the reason I practiced positive self-talk. Here are some parts of my recordings:

"Heather, you are magnetic; you are beautiful; you're kind and loving, successful and smart"

When you grow older, usually you don't hear these words from others, so you may need to repeat them for yourself. When I started recording, these sentences were so foreign to me, but now I look forward to hearing them; this is my self-hypnosis, in a way.

5. Somatic Experience

I also enjoy somatic experiencing exercises because they are very fast and easy; only 20-30 seconds a couple of times a day can completely change your nervous system and how you show up. They help your nervous system shift out of that fight-or-flight mode and into rest, digest, and heal, without having to relive the trauma that caused the problem in the first place. What?!? How awesome is that!

6. Other Self-care methods

You can also try following self-care methods:

a. Breath work

b. Tapping

c. Getting natural vitamin D

I lay out in the sun for 20 minutes every day with my feet on the ground as I'm meditating. A lot of times if you can combine certain modalities together. That makes the treatments a little more efficient. So, that way, I'm grounding to recharge my body system and get some of those negative ions from the earth and disperse some of these EMFs (Electro-Magnetic Field Theory) that we're constantly bombarded with. The earth is like a battery for us; when we put our bare feet on the ground, we recharge our bodies. So, I'm recharging and getting my vitamin D and meditating all at the same time; that is my supercharger technique.

Last Words

If you are at a point in your life where you have been diagnosed with an autoimmune disease, you can stay on that pill, or that injection, or whatever other band-aid they throw at you, for the rest of your life. Or I would love for you to get rid of that paradigm and understand that is absolutely possible to heal and lessen, if not reverse, your symptoms. I was pleasantly surprised when I was able to reverse two out of my three autoimmune diseases.

Look at the different areas in your life that you could improve. Little steps add up over time! Let's do a challenge. Can you remove toxins from your body or from your environment? Can you change your mindset? Can you change your shopping list and eat healthier food or filtered water? Can you change when you go to bed? These are the areas of health you must investigate if you want long-lasting health; the kind of health that gives you the energy to explore this beautiful world, play with your kids and grandchildren, dance, hike, and go on adventures; the kind that helps you experience joy in your life and peace in your body; a brain that works and a body that doesn't hurt. No matter how common a symptom, maybe it is NEVER normal. You deserve to thrive, not just survive.

Find a guide who can help you on your journey. You don't have to do it alone. Are you ready to take your first step? I can help. I have been where you are. I understand what you are going through.

CHAPTER 5: The Secrets of Longevity; Can We Control Our DNA?

By Kellie Lupsha, Women's Longevity Expert

In 2006, I dropped my kids (one and four years old at the time) off at daycare very early in the morning and headed to work. I was working as the Director of Therapy for a rehabilitation hospital. Another day of busyness and exhaustion. The furthest thing from my mind was creating a life of longevity. Honestly, I was just surviving, until later that day I got "the call." It was my mom calling to tell me, my dad was just diagnosed with cancer. I was in total shock, thinking this could not be. I knew he had more life to live, for himself and my mom, as well as with me and my brother, my children and even my grandchildren.

I had a privilege of growing up with all my grandparents and most of my great-grandparents, so it never crossed my mind that my kids might not experience the same. So many thoughts were racing through my head, like… my dad had no family history of cancer, we were relatively healthy, well… he was overweight, he did lead a stressful life, he didn't have an outlet for stress relief, he probably could have exercised and eaten better. But still, cancer! He died three years later. I was devastated. My kids never experienced my dad as their grandfather. His passing made me begin to question health and medicine as I knew it. I never imagined he would die so young.

My Story

I have been in the health and wellness industry for over 25 years as a physical therapist and a women's longevity coach. My husband and I both have specialized in helping people all over the world recover from neurological disorders, such as traumatic brain injuries, strokes, and concussions. We have been blessed to help so many individuals and families in these difficult times to regain their lives. Through our time working with clients, we realized that it was more than just physical therapy that they needed in their journey to recovery.

Our patients really needed help on a cellular level: cleaning up their cells, optimizing their genes, and supporting nutrition so their brain and body could have the proper support to recover even more. We decided to dig into the research ourselves, since many of the practitioners just wanted to keep adding more drugs to our patient's regime. We knew there must be a better way.

I began to 'learn, seek, and question' every aspect of what I thought I already knew. As I shared earlier, my father had passed away at 69 of lymphoma, leaving me very perplexed as to where his cancer came from, as he had no family history of cancer. Was this really his fate? Could he have prevented this? Was there a lifestyle component? So, I went on a quest to answer these questions. What I found is we control more of our body and our genes! We discovered the power of both functional and longevity medicine and the field of Nutrigenomics.

The science behind functional and longevity medicine is based on years of scientific discovery. Thank you to so many pioneers, such as Dr. Jeffery Bland, Dr. Mark Hyman, Dr. David Sinclair, Dr. Peter Diamandis, Dr. David Perlmutter, and so many more for paving the way. The future of technology looks promising and exhilarating in wellness and longevity. Over the past 10 years, we have experienced amazing results and wonderful personal stories applying this science to our family, patients and clients.

I once believed my fate was in the genes inherited from my family and I too would be diagnosed with breast cancer, just like my maternal grandmother. According to 2022 statistics from http://breastcancer.org, one in eight women will be diagnosed with breast cancer in her lifetime. Therefore, from a young age, I feared I would be diagnosed with breast cancer too. Since then, I have learned that's the furthest from the truth. I will share more about the story of my genes later in this chapter.

Our Daughter's Asthma

I began studying the field of functional medicine and using nutrigenomics to activate genes and apply it to my family members. Our oldest daughter had a long history of asthma, which impacted her life significantly throughout her teen years. She needed to make sure she had her inhaler everywhere she went. She often found herself using it many times a day and was also taking additional medications to manage her asthma at the time. Her asthma impacted many aspects of her daily life. Struggling to breathe can affect all activities, including schoolwork, extracurricular activities, and just being a kid with her friends. She was frustrated about needing to rely on her medications so much that, at times, it even affected her mood and social interactions.

When we started making changes to her diet and lifestyle as well as activate her genes, she was able to make the transition off her medication. The other day she told me, "Mom, I do not even remember the last time I used my inhaler." It has been a gift sharing how to take control of her health with her and instilling these beliefs for her future longevity.

Our Youngest Daughter's Migraines

Our youngest child ended up with a concussion on her 10th birthday and then with severe migraines. On several occasions, she presented as if she was experiencing a neurological event like a stroke or even a brain tumor. However, all the tests thankfully came back negative. But one time, I was called into the nurse's office at her school. As I arrived, she didn't recognize me, couldn't speak, and had difficulty moving. At that moment, I thought for sure she was having a massive seizure or stroke. We immediately called 9-1-1. Of course, for the first year of her episodes, no one could figure out what was happening to her After all the diagnostic testing on her last admission, still no answers. After ruling everything else out, her pediatrician came back stating these events she was having must be migraines. The symptoms she experienced, which usually began with an aura that came on prior to the migraine; as a result, she had lost her ability to feel on one side and her ability to speak. As a medical practitioner, I didn't even realize that the symptoms were neurologically induced by a migraine. Even after getting a diagnosis, our doctors didn't have answers for us. Their solution was, when the event occurs, to get her to a quiet place and take this medicine. At that point, we knew we needed to take our family's health into our own hands.

After we realized the impact of changing managing stress, modifying diet and lifestyle, activating her genes, and gut health and got her body back in balance just like for our eldest daughter too. If I could help my own family, I could help so many more people, teaching them that they are in control of their genes and their destiny. We can all have the potential to live long and thrive. I am happy to say, my daughter has not experienced these migraines now in over five years after being activated through nutrigenomics and implementing lifestyle and nutrition changes.

The Ultimate Goal: Prevention versus Treatment

When we are talking about prevention, no matter what our genetic blueprint, there are a handful of things we should all be doing to aid in optimal wellness, including sleep, downtime, breathwork, nutrition, and movement. I am not going to go in depth on any of those specifically, but I can't just dismiss the fact that we need to briefly talk about each one.

Sleep. Good sleep is critical. What is "good" sleep? You may be thinking, "I go to bed every day and get 7–8 hours of sleep, so I'm good, what else is there to talk about?" Sleep is more than sleep; the health benefits are immense, probably more than you have even imagined. We need to work on and develop a sleep routine to have quality sleep, where our body goes through the four stages of sleep for approximately five cycles. Each cycle is an average of 90 minutes. For some individuals, it may be as long as120 minutes and for others only 75 minutes. Therefore, the time we need to sleep varies for each of us. What doesn't vary in the need for deep and REM sleep. Let me bust the myth, right now, that some of you can actually function on 4–5 hours of sleep. It may seem like that today, but I can guarantee that your body is not repairing and replenishing your cells, which in turn may lead you to age faster. It is in the deep restorative sleep that our DNA repairs, our cells clean out the trash, and we boost our immune system. When we sleep according to our unique needs, our bodies can function optimally, so we can start the day off well, restored and energized. Conversely, if we do not achieve quality sleep, our bodies accelerate aging, which may in turn lead to dysfunction and ultimately to "dis–ease" (lack of ease or comfort leading to imbalances at the cellular level), or even disease.

The Importance of Downtime "Active Rest"

Just like sleep, our bodies repair with rest. Many of us have found ourselves constantly multitasking and overloading our brains and bodies. Unfortunately, this leads to early aging. It is critical for each one of us to make sure that we are building our health foundation with rest, stopping the cycles of stress and burnout. Our stressors may go away, but we must help our bodies actually complete the stress cycle. Incorporating stress reduction techniques, enjoying downtime, and having relaxation, laughing, enjoying hobbies are essential to breaking that stress cycle.

I'll be honest, I used to believe that rest was for lazy people. "I was so wrong." It is easy for all of us to become caught with the business of life. Unfortunately, the level of 'go-go-go' we all feel creates more stress, leading to damage of our cells, creating chaos and ultimately oxidative stress. This is one of reasons why illness, chronic disease, autoimmune disorders, and cancers are on the rise.

For the busy ones amongst us, it is so easy to just say, "I did my yoga, I did my gratitude," and check it off the box. I want you to think, "It is not about the list, and it is not about checking off the box; it is about you." Ask yourself, "Am I fully allowing myself to reset? Am I giving myself the grace of this downtime to rest and restore? Am I building up my health, so I don't end up in the stress and burnout cycle?" If not, this is where your genes may decide to misbehave, where you may begin suppressing (turning off) your positive or good genes and expressing (turning on) your negative or bad genes. Your health is truly under your control.

We now know from clinicians and research institutions, like Dr. Mark Hyman and 3X4 Genetics, that approximately 4–8% of our genes are hard-wired. Our lifestyle choices control the other 92–96%. Therefore, even if you have a family history of diabetes or cancer, it is no longer your fate. You are in control. You can become the CEO of your health. Later in this chapter, we will discuss further how to optimize your genes and take more control of your health.

Breathing and Breathwork

I will readily admit, I am not an expert in breathwork; however, I know the simple blessing of breath is essential in creating longevity. Through my time as an athlete, a physical therapist, a mom, and now women's longevity coach, I have learned that breathing is an important part of wellness in every aspect of life. Over time, many of us begin to breathe shallowly, or start mouth breathing, leading to a poor influence on our health.

In Chapter 3 of *The Gap* https:/acechoiceidea.com/funnel/the-gap/, Dr. Nayman describes the effects of poor breathing as well as the benefits of breathwork and several breathing exercises. Go back for your reference. It is extensive. I have always worked on my breathing, even before I knew it was so essential for my health. A few years ago, I had the pleasure of experiencing two transformational breathwork sessions that assisted me in breaking through blocks in my life holding me back. I had no idea breathwork could be that powerful. Today, I practice box breathing for my usual breathwork when I'm stressed, as well as when I'm relaxing in the infrared sauna.

Breathing is essential to life; however, throughout our lives, this natural process often becomes disrupted. Learning to breathe and having breath work is something that we often forget, and we can take it for granted, like sleep. As a specialist with brain disorders, I know the link between breath and brain activity. We all need oxygen delivery and exchange in all our tissues. The benefits are immense and necessary. Whether you are looking to improve your sleep or your athletic performance, boost your immunity, improve your mood, or just feel more energized, just begin the basics of breathwork. A great place to start is just close your mouth and become aware of your breathing, begin to feel and experience your breath. If you need more go to YouTube and search breathing or box breathing techniques. However, if you are serious about learning more, I agree with Dr. Nayman, in her recommendation of the book *Breath*, by James Nestor.

Food is Information

Nutrition is absolutely a key to building our foundation of health. We used to say that smoking was one of the worst things you could do for your health, but honestly, eating certain foods, like trans fats, is probably even more dangerous than smoking. I am in no way promoting smoking! However, as smoking is bad, imagine trans fats are worse! I hope by now you have realized there is nothing healthy about eating most fast foods. If you've jumped on the diet fads, we must realize all fads will come and go. We need to eat for health.

So, what should we eat, not eat, how should we eat? It can be confusing. Let's begin with eating real, whole foods. The first step is to clean up food intake by eliminating prepackaged, processed, and boxed foods. This is where we find so many ingredients that we cannot even pronounce are hidden, like additives, chemicals, toxins, and more. Our bodies often reject these ingredients, storing them as toxins in our fat cells. Think about what most people ate before the convenience of mega grocery stores: people bought fresh fruits and vegetables from the local farmer, fresh meat and fish from the butcher, and fresh bread from the bakers. There were no preservatives, pesticides, or chemicals in our foods. Now, in the 21st century, our foods are full of artificial colors, flavors, additives, preservatives, GMOs, and more. Our bodies may react as these foreign substances are invaders and are causing alerts and creating inflammation.

Food is information. It tells our cells to perform or not to perform certain processes. Eat the food that is going to fuel your body. Consider eating a wide variety of organic, non-GMO fruits and vegetables. Eat a variety of grass-fed and finished meats, wild caught and sustainable fish. Consume nutrient-dense carbohydrates in moderation. Keep your sugars, gluten, and dairy low, or even eliminate them, as they are inflammatory.

Food is the baseline for your health, and it also helps prevent disease. The next time you take a bite of food or order from a restaurant, ask yourselves, "Will this fuel my cells? Am I providing energy or taking away energy from my body?" Then make the best choice. Life is full of choices and constantly striving for perfection may lead us to fail. I always ask myself, "What is my best option at the time?" This allows me to enjoy food, go out with others and be in community, and keep my body as happy as possible. Just FYI, I avoid gluten and dairy, and I am still able to find options so I can eat out and have fun, as well as have enjoyment cooking and eating at home. So, enjoy your food in honor of your health.

Move Your Body

With my background of 25 years of being a physical therapist, I need to share the importance of movement. For myself, I knew at a young age I needed to move, and I enjoyed moving. Our bodies were meant to move. As we move, walk, stretch, and bend, we bring in blood supply and nutrients to our joints, muscles, and organs, including our brain. We provide benefits to our heart and lungs with brisk activity. We provide our brain and nervous system with chemicals to support our mental health. Moderate daily exercise is essential. Our bodies also need the proper stressors to activate our longevity genes, keep our muscles strong to support ourselves, and maintain flexibility to keep moving and be active throughout life. We once thought our bodies required 60–90 minutes of exercises; fortunately, new research shows, 5–20 minutes of intensity may be all you need. No more excuses of, "I don't have time."

Please listen to this: Without movement, we will not age well. Finding an activity that you enjoy is extremely important because it will inspire and encourage you to move. If you force yourself to follow a specific program which you do not really enjoy, then it won't last; just like "dieting" you will give up easily or find an excuse to postpone or discontinue. Think of movement as life. Find an activity that you can do at least three to five times a week and mix it up with activities that support your brain, heart, lungs, and muscles/joints. Think about 10 minutes of strenuous activity followed by stretching in the morning and a 10-minute brisk walk after dinner. It will not only give you the benefits above but also support your metabolic health, too. So, get moving!

What is Your Customized Lifestyle plan?

What we previously talked about are typical lifestyle components that will generally keep us healthier: Sleep, downtime, breathing/breathwork, nutrition, and movement. Now we need to discover what we can do to uniquely tailor our lifestyle to our own body. We can't answer this question until we really look at our DNA. Let's start with a few terms. A person's genotype is their unique sequence of DNA. Phenotype is the detectable expression of the genotype (a person's clinical presentation, how they look).

Some of you may be saying to yourself, "No thank you, I'd rather not know what my genes say," and others of you are getting excited right now, thinking, "I can take more control of my health." I was scared at first, thinking, "Do I really want to know what is in my genes?" However, knowing my genes were not my fate, I knew I needed to know so I could take more control of my health. My lifestyle choices will determine how my genes act. It has been said by many in the functional medicine field that our genes may load the gun. However, it is our lifestyle choices that pull the trigger. Therefore, if I can have a road map according to my unique DNA, then I can avoid or decrease my risk of my genes turning on or off. Get it? I wouldn't accidentally pull the trigger.

As I said earlier, my maternal grandmother had breast cancer, so I thought I would too. Even though I regularly exercise and eat healthy food, I believed I would still end up with breast cancer. I had it in my mind for years until I did all my genetic testing. I was excited to find out that the specific breast cancer gene for me is low penetrance (a low risk of turning on or being expressed). At the same time, I was shocked to find out which genes I have that are high penetrance (a high risk of turning on or a high likelihood of being expressed).

Let me back up and explain more about the penetrance of genes.

The penetrance (impact) refers to how likely a person is to show a specific physical trait based on their genetic blueprint. High penetrance relates to genetic changes that are powerful and impactful with an increased chance of impacting our biochemistry. In high penetrance, our genes play a significant role and our environment and the daily choice we make (epigenetics) has a lesser role. Low penetrance is the opposite, where our environment and daily choices we make have a far more significant impact on our health and the individual gene variants by themselves play a lesser role. That doesn't mean we ignore the gene, but rather focus on the right daily choices.

To further explain penetrance, follow my analogy. Let's say you need to get to your closest major airport. In a perfect route, there would be nothing major in your way; no traffic, road construction, or poor weather to slow you down. This is the best scenario: Just like if you had a no-impact gene, or a low-impact gene, there is nothing in your way. However, as we see the increase in gene penetrance from low to medium, high, and very high, getting to the airport is more difficult. You may experience more traffic, or road construction that slows you down, or even closed exits or complete roadblocks. In any of these examples, knowing the roadblocks allows us to reroute and build an alternative route. We will still arrive at the airport, just on a different path.

This is what we can create for you, your unique blueprint. By knowing your unique DNA, you can create customized routes for you with food and nutrients, exercise, rest, and more, that are based on your genes.

Most DNA tests tell which genes you have. What is often missing is the penetrance of the genes and how genes work in pathways. To share more of my story, one of my high penetrance genes is HLA DQ2.5/DQ2.5. This is the celiac gene, which I acquired from both of my parents. If you are familiar with celiac disease, most people who have it are very sick. It is a long-term autoimmune disorder primarily affecting the small intestine. For me, this gene has not been expressed or turned on, even though I have a very high risk of turning it on. I now know this is a major roadblock. Therefore, to avoid it, I will remain gluten and dairy free as well as manage my inflammatory and oxidative stress pathways to keep that gene suppressed (turned off).

Here is more on pathways. Besides looking at penetrance of genes, looking at them as pathways versus individual genes is very helpful at determining genetic susceptibility. Pathway analysis involves taking a series of low penetrance genes and grouping them together, so they form a stronger and more precise picture of an individual's genetic susceptibility. A few examples of a pathway include the pathway of oxidative stress, detoxification, memory, and brain health.

Two of the pathways I need to manage are my inflammatory pathway and my oxidative stress pathway. The inflammatory pathway is protective by design, but it can become destructive if left unchecked, leading to chronic disease. The oxidative stress pathway is like human rusting. The impact of all exposures over time results in damage to our cells. If this pathway is unmanaged, oxidative stress can impact our energy levels, memory, premature aging, and even increase cancer risk. To bring this full circle, even though when looking at my breast cancer gene in isolation the penetrance is low, if my pathways of inflammation and oxidative stress are not managed, my breast cancer gene may become expressed (turned on) even though on its own, it is of low risk to me.

I love to teach people that you can be the CEO of your health; you are in charge, and if you know your road map, Your DNA Blueprint, of what you need to do and where your detours are, not only you can make it there, but you can live an extraordinary long and healthy life.

Genome, Epigenome, and Nutrigenomics

Your genome is made up of an identical instruction set of 3.2 billion letters from your mother and father. These letters make up your DNA and are known as your genome. Your epigenome is the cellular software that controls your DNA, your genome, telling it to turn on or off. If you imagine your genes being the keys of a piano, your epigenome is the piano player. Your epigenome is involved in regulating gene expression. The epigenome can be dynamically altered by environmental conditions and your lifestyle choices. You are the piano player; you are in charge of what your genes are going to say (how they express). Your solutions to build a strong health foundation are in your control. So how do we do it?

The first part of the solution is how to customize your lifestyle to your unique DNA needs. We need to build a solution that is unique to each one of us, whether it's sleep, how we detox, how we methylate[24].

[24] revolutionaryhealth.com: Methylation is a chemical reaction that occurs in every cell and tissue in your body. In some instances, methylation of proteins helps the body detoxify. For example, the

The second part of the solution is to minimize or eliminate stressors. Environmental pollutants, toxins, benzenes, EMFs, and so many more chemicals make our bodies work harder than they should, at times even harder than we are capable of sustaining.

This is one of the reasons we are seeing chronic disease and autoimmune disorders on the rise, both in adults and children. Therefore, our genes may need a bit more help than years ago. These environmental stressors may start to turn our genes on or off much earlier in our life compared to 100 years ago. Evaluate your environment to see what you can change to optimize your family's health. Ensure that you check household products, from skin and hair products to carpet and mattresses. Negative chemicals and toxins can be found everywhere. Seek out a full resource guide at https://www.ewg.org/consumer-guides or through the app Think Dirty[25].

---

methylation process helps convert a toxic amino acid (homocysteine) into a beneficial amino acid (methionine)*) or how we metabolize caffeine, salt, or vitamin D. The list can go on and on, but once you know you can build that plan to optimize your genes. I highly suggest having a practitioner guide you in understanding your DNA results. Not all DNA tests are the same. And not all DNA tests provide user friendly information. * Defined by revolutionaryhealth.com

[25] Think Dirty – Shop Clean on the App Store (apple.com)

The good news is we can optimize our genes using nutrigenomics. "Nutrigenomics is the study of how foods interact with your genes and explains the individual genetic differences that can affect the requirements of vitamins, minerals, and compounds in the foods we eat.[26]" Nutrigenomics is one of the most exciting, revolutionary, and cutting-edge fields in nutrition, genetics, and modern wellness. This field uses a combination of nutrition and natural ingredients and how they interact with our metabolic process to activate our genes. This means no matter what your DNA says, the goal is to keep your good/positive genes working well and your bad/negative genes turned down or even off. Nutrigenomics is becoming a powerhouse in turning on essential protein pathways needed for longevity. To learn more about pathways, you can refer to Appendix.

How Can We Grow Older Gracefully?

What we know now is to get started making changes today. The future is bright, but you need to stay on top of your health to catch this wave of science and technology coming with an explosion of longevity tools. If you don't, you may be too late to take advantage of what is coming in the future of health and wellness.

---

[26] https://nutritiongenome.com

Let me ask you, when you think about aging, what is the picture you paint in your mind? Do you see someone who's frail, in a wheelchair, maybe in a nursing home needing help? Or do you see a person who is walking on the beach, gardening and traveling, and playing with their grandchildren or even great-grandchildren? Living long into old age no longer must mean being sick in a nursing home. We can all age gracefully with the knowledge and technology that is available today. We can live in vitality and with tons of energy throughout our lives. People think that longevity is in the future, but in fact, longevity is the potential of aging gracefully now.

A few key takeaways that we talked about earlier in this chapter are in prevention and understanding your unique DNA blueprint. You are perfectly positioned to get started on your longevity journey today, with exercise and nutrition, intermittent fasting and not eating too much, watching how you eat, going back to whole foods and decreasing stress, eliminating burnout and busyness, and building a sleep routine! You can also choose to become the CEO of your own health and purse, discovering the lifestyle for your unique DNA. If you look at a variety of places around the world where longevity is happening, it is the blue zones like Japan, Italy, Greece, Costa Rica, Nicoya, Ikaria, and Loma Linda, California. We now have the knowledge to create the model of longevity for ourselves, our families, and our communities.

Following the Common Path is Not the Answer

By now I hope you understand the quality of your life is the quality of your cells. When you look at and follow what is common, chances are you'll end up aging poorly, since that is currently very common. I know at times it is difficult to step outside the norm, as we all have needs to be seen, heard, and celebrated. When you change, that same group may not be celebrating your changes and they may even want to challenge you to just stay the same. When we act and think differently, we may get teased, ignored, or even ridiculed. I challenge you to step outside your comfort zone, show others you are going to take control of your health and be the role model for yourself, your family, and others to see what is possible if we step outside of average or common. This will require many of you to change your lifestyle and your behaviors, and maybe even your community. It had been said by many, we become the average of five people we surround ourselves with the most. So, I ask you, who are you surrounding yourself with? If you feel there isn't a community for you, you're wrong; between books, podcasts, and online groups, there are plenty of us cheering you on. Find your tribe.

Last Words

I am excited to tell you, you no longer need to worry about a life of frailty and sickness because you have the power to create the life of longevity and thrive. I am asking you to take action, choose to live an extraordinary life. There are simple steps to get started; pick one area to focus on and gradually add another step. Choose to believe you are healthy and decide to live that life. Create a plan for sleep and rest to fit your needs. Maximize your longevity with your food and nutrition. Build movement into your life. Keep your mind right on both the basics of prevention and on living a lifestyle according to your unique DNA blueprint to truly live a life in longevity.

CHAPTER 6: How A Little Change in My Mom's Lifestyle Saved Her Life

By Betty Khalili, Registered Nurse, and Bestselling Author

As a registered nurse working for more than two decades, I can't bear seeing any member of my family suffer from chronic pain. A little tweak in our lifestyle can easily reverse most chronic disease. Working and recommending lifestyle changes to my patients made me confident that I can help my family members do the same.

My mom suffered from terrible regurgitation attacks almost every two weeks. She had tried any treatment she knew, any prescribed pill from well-known medical doctors, and different diet styles. Everyone in our family was concerned while watching her retching and barfing her stomach contents out and throwing up bile at the end. It was so heartbreaking looking at her fragile, pale face when she moaned and wished herself dead over these pains. We took her to the emergency room very often. They gave her injections (antiemetic and anti-cramps) and an intravenous fluid. Her fragile skin did not allow nurses to get a proper IV set. Each time, they poked her frail skin multiple times, and she came home bruised on her hands and arms. I had been sending her new medications for years. She had tried almost all of them, but with little effect. Every phone call to her, hearing her painful voice, was heart-wrenching for me. I was at the end of the rope with my help. Nothing seemed to be working. In her endoscopy, the report emphasized varicose veins in her esophagus[27]. Her esophagus was narrow and inflamed, with a lot of redness at its edges. The valve between her stomach and esophagus had been dilated and the stomach acid traveled up and made it worse. She had had enough, and we were all disappointed and frustrated that we could not help her anymore. I was afraid, knowing all the side effects of long-term use of all those drugs and not being sure much longer she was going to need them. Those medications may have led her to early Alzheimer's, dementia, and many more problems….

I read a lot, investigated non-stop, and consulted with our physicians in ICU and each of my friends' physician. One night I sat and wrote down all I had gathered in a summary and planned a lifestyle change for Mom. Knowing her and every tiny detail in her lifestyle helped me a lot. I collected what I knew and researched

[27] Barrett's esophagus - Symptoms and causes - Mayo Clinic

over the years and wrote down the program for her. I sent it to my brothers, and called them and explained every step, emphasizing that each tiny note is important. One of my brothers jotted down the program on papers with big fonts and gave it to her. She hung the paper on the wall and reminded herself every day to go through it and follow it. One month later, she told me: "None of these well-known doctors could cure me for years. Your plan saved me, and I feel much better now. I don't have the stomach aches, cramps, and nausea/vomiting anymore."

I was thrilled to hear that; tears of joy and honor were flowing down my face. It has been more than three years now, and I'm beyond excited to announce that she has not taken any pill for her pain for more than three years and she hasn't experienced the symptoms anymore. I concluded that all that suffering was not only because of her diet and what she ate. There were a lot of components, especially her lifestyle and mindset, attached to her health issues.

What did I observe?

I decided to go through her daily life and how she managed her daily activities. In Islam, when we do prayers, it requires bending a few times and staying in that position for a long time. My Mom is religious and does the prayers five times a day. She did her prayers right after each meal. I also figured out she laid down and slept after prayer. We went through the time when she had the worst pain.

She had heartburn and regurgitation immediately after praying and after waking up following each meal.

She used to drink water during her meal and that worsened her situation.

We decided to go through a plan for her from the moment she woke up until she went to bed. She had to follow every step very carefully.

Food Categorization in Persian Culture and How to Balance the Food

Before discussing Mom's plan, I would like to introduce our way of categorizing foods. In Persian culture, we divide food into two groups: cold and warm. I am not talking about the temperature but the nature of the food, meaning that some foods have the nature of being cold and need more work to digest, like yogurt, raw vegetables, and red meat. The warm foods are full of calories and energy, and they are easier to assimilate. Consuming too much cold food will cause headaches, mess up your stomach, and trigger diarrhea; in contrary, warm foods have an irritating effect on your body, and especially initiate rashes and itchiness on your skin if they are consumed in large amounts. In traditional Persian cooking, we mix warm and cold foods to neutralize the extreme effect of the warm or cold nature. For example, we have a traditional dish called *Fessenjan*. It's a delicious stew with pomegranate paste, walnut, and meat. Pomegranate is cold in nature and walnut is warm. We mix them to neutralize the natures.

Word of Caution

Some foods and fruits may have an inflammatory effect on you. They make you suffer from headaches, gaining weight, migraines, or heartburn. Over years, our body might react to some particular foods. Your customized diet plan might be toxic for someone else.

We basically don't notice this inflammatory response because it happens so slowly in the long run. It manifests itself in the form of various diseases such as migraine, arthritis, eczema, depression, inflammation, gut, stomach, and intestinal discomfort, and even cancer.

The Importance of Taking a Food Sensitivity Test

I always recommend doing a food sensitivity test which tells you exactly which foods you are sensitive to. Here I tried to create a generic plan which almost fits everyone, but you need to know your own customized needs. You might be sensitive to tomato, mango, or something you are really not aware of.

I personally found out that I have sensitivity to pistachio; I get some itchiness and rashes right away after consumption. When I did my food sensitivity test, the status for pistachios was in a red zone. Since I was a kid, I was raised in a place where we had a pistachio garden, and we ate pistachios in large amounts. The reaction got worse over the years. Now I try to avoid eating pistachios, or I may have one or two at a time to satisfy the temptation.

If a certain food makes you sick, remove it from your diet.

I read a book called *The Plan* from Lyn-genet[28]. It helped me understand how to create a custom food plan for my mom and for myself. Lyn-genet wrote the book by studying thousands of people. The author showed that a series of foods cause an inflammatory reaction in 80% of people and grouped them according to the intensity of their reaction. In this book, another way to recognize reactive foods is to clean the body for 20 days; then we introduce

---

[28] https:/www.amazon.com/dp/B007ZGBX5I/

one food at a time to see the reaction the next day by weighing ourselves and taking our body temperature.

My Mom's Lifestyle Plan

Here are the instructions I wrote down for my mom's diet in sequential order, from the time she wakes up until she goes to bed, based on my research and applying it on my patients.

1. When you wake up in the morning, you start your day with a glass of warm water with some lemon juice and fresh ginger in it.

2. Wait half an hour to one hour before having your breakfast.

3. Avoid using any cow products because your experiences talk to you. You have a stomach-ache after consuming cow products; so, go dairy-free.

4. Limit taking wheat-based bread.

5. Consume tea without sugar. You can substitute sugar with dates, dried figs, or raisins.

6. I recommend intermittent fasting. Do not eat for two to three hours before lunch.

7. For lunch you can have baked chicken or fish; no cow products are allowed, only sheep or goat products. You can eat rice with your meat.

8. No liquid is allowed during the meal. Take room temperature water half an hour before or after each meal. You need to keep your body hydrated with at least 2-2.5 liters per day. Lack of water causes drying of body tissues and organs and inflammatory reactions. Excessive consumption of water causes retention of water in cells and increases weight.

9. Do your prayers before a big meal and avoid physical activities after the meal. I recommend doing your prayer in a standing or sitting position.

10. No lying down is allowed until one hour after each meal.

11. Eat in peace, take time to taste and chew your food slowly.

12. Stop worrying or thinking about your problems while eating.

13. Consume vegetables either steamed, oven baked, or roasted, and not raw. Vegetables such as broccoli, carrots, spinach, and celery should not be eaten raw. Vegetables like potatoes may need a little more time to cook.

14. For dinner, you can have fruit that goes well with your stomach, chosen by experience and season.

15. Stop eating at 7 p.m., three hours before you go to bed.

16. Eat organic and avoid processed and canned products. If you want to buy tomato paste, buy it in glass containers and not in cans.

17. Avoid overcooking eggs and meat since their protein molecules will break down and cause inflammation.

18. Substitute saturated fats with unsaturated fats such as olive oil and avocado to prevent heart attack and stroke. Omega-3 fatty acid boosts heart health by improving cholesterol levels, lowering blood clotting, lessening irregular heartbeats, and slightly decreasing blood pressure[29].

19. Use Sea salt instead of other manufactured salt. While cooking, add a very small amount of salt and use more turmeric, saffron, black pepper, paprika, fresh ginger root, garlic, onion, and parsley.

Last Words

You can't imagine how a little tweak in your lifestyle can relieve you of years of pain and suffering. For people who are suffering

[29] Dietary fat: Know which to choose - Mayo Clinic

from GI symptoms, I believe the best help is to create a diary of your habits before, during, and after a big meal.

Do you drink cold water? Do you drink it right before or after your meal?

What do you do right after your meal? Do you sleep or take exercise immediately after your meal?

What do you feel once you finish eating each meal? Are you bloated and gassy? Does your stomach get upset after eating or drinking a certain food?

Do you take time to eat, or you are playing with your cellphone, watching stressful news, or thinking about your problems in your household or at work?

By connecting mind and body, we can be more aware of our health status. We are not the slave of food; we can wisely control what we eat and how we treat our body.

CHAPTER 7: Some Fun and Healthy Recipes

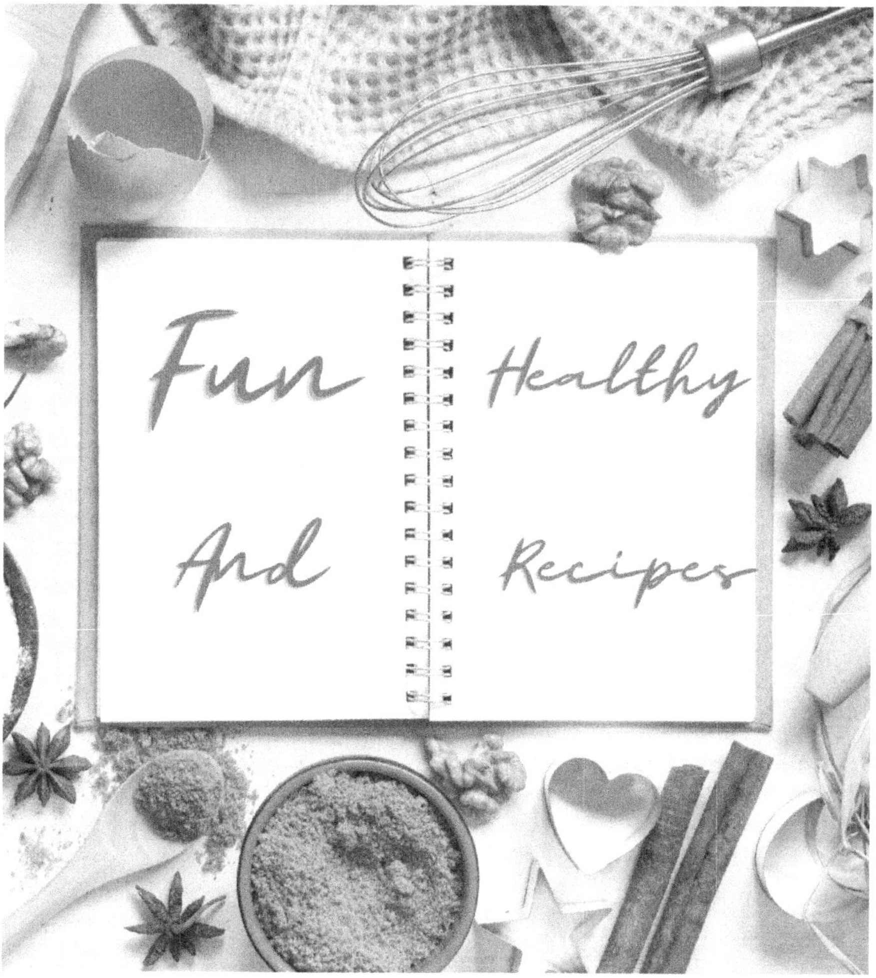

Filet and Veggies by Reed Davis

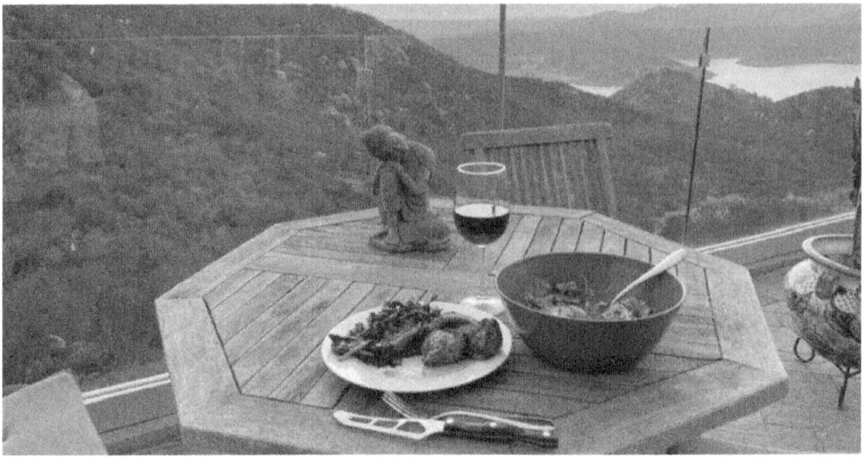

Always purchase the best quality, grass-fed, grass-finished filet mignon you can find. You can often get a good deal on the "tenderloin tails" and they grill quite nicely. I buy from my local butcher but ordering online works too. Look up Certified Piedmontese. The main reason everyone loves my grilling starts with the quality of meat!

Beef should be at room temperature, marinated as you please. I use "Coco Aminos" as it is gluten-free. Sprinkle on your favorite seasonings, mix it up, and cover so it can sit for a little while. This is where you get to be creative, but the biggest mistake you can make is to over-salt. Your job is to provide perfectly grilled and flavorful meat and let your guests salt to taste.

A nice hot grill is important to sear in the flavor and juices. Grill for just a few minutes on each side to the desired temperature. I've served hundreds of guests and you can never go wrong with *medium*. Nice and juicy and pink.

Slicing and serving is very important. Use a large cutting board and invest in a professional chef's knife for slicing your meat. At my table, I slice the steaks up perfectly so my guests can take what they want off the cutting board. Mmmm… warm and juicy.

For the veggies, I usually throw them in a pan with olive oil and garlic. You can play with adding some butter or ghee or coconut oil if you like the added flavor. My advantage here is that I grow my own vegetables and can pick what's ripe, straight from the garden. If you are interested in growing your own veggies, check out Lettuce Grow, a self-watering, self-fertilizing hydroponic farmstand. They'll ship you everything you need to grow on your porch or even inside.

As I said, put a little oil in the pan with some fresh chopped garlic. When it's hot you can start adding your veggies, such as asparagus, broccolini, spinach, etc. Add some sliced organic mushrooms to the hot oil and garlic if you like, and any favorite seasoning or condiment. Once it gets going, remember to turn the temperature down so you don't burn your pan (or ruin the garlic).

Serve food hot if possible. Put meat on a large cutting board per above and dump your pan of hot veggies into a nice serving dish so folks can help themselves. Add some seeds or herbs on top if you want to get fancy. A nice wine or cold kombucha is popular in my house and sure to please almost company. Of course, one could add a nice fresh salad and homemade dressing to make this recipe a complete meal.

Grilling and stove-top cooking should be quick and easy with minimal cleanup. Do it as a couple! Starting with a clean kitchen makes it easy to keep track of everything.

Enjoy!

Reed Davis

Fruity Breakfast by Pantea Kalhor

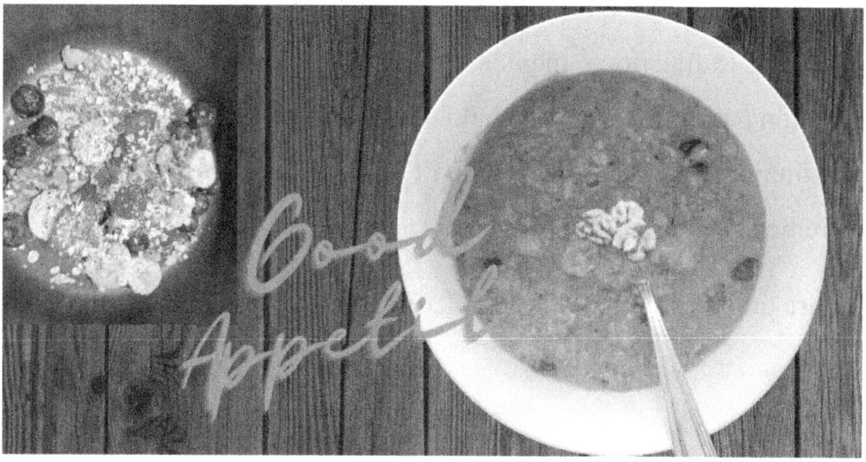

My clients ask me, “Okay, if we remove bread, cheese, and dairy products, what can we eat for breakfast?” That may be a question especially for a typical Persian family, as we all get used to eating dairy products, milk, and cheese for breakfast. Oatmeal Fruity Breakfast was my favorite choice while going through healing and I still prepare it in the morning.

Word of caution

Did you know all of us may be sensitive to some foods which we are not aware of? Sometimes we force ourselves to eat something because of its benefits, not knowing we can be allergic to it. Those certain foods can bring us inflammation. If you are bloating after eating certain foods or have some digestion issues, a food sensitivity test can help you discover more about what you can eat and what you can't. In functional medicine, we design a specific nutrition plan based on patients' complaints and health history and their body constitution. I assume that you don't have any allergy to the ingredients I brought here.

Before proceeding to our recipe, let's answer some questions.

True or False

Myth: Having seasonal salad as dinner is a great choice!!

Answer: A mix of lotus, cucumber, and tomato is very cold in nature, which needs lots of energy to digest. In case you still like to consume it, use some walnut to give a warmer nature to the salad. However, we suggest eating steamed vegetables such as carrot, cauliflower, and broccoli to warm up your stomach and help digestion.

Myth: By cutting carbohydrates from our diet, we can lose weight and stay healthy.

Answer: Carbohydrates cannot be completely removed from your diet as we need them to get energy and balance our diet. However, we recommend a more gluten-free diet and removing white wheat bread from your diet.

My Favorite Fruity Breakfast Recipe

Ingredients:

1 c. Ground Flax seed

1 Tbsp. Hempseed

3-4 pieces of Walnut

1 1/2 c. Almond Milk (you can the homemade recipe here, however, I use it unsweet)

1 small Banana

1 c. mixed berries (I usually add blueberry and blackberry)

In the main recipe, I used to include some oatmeal. However, since oatmeal may trigger autoimmune disease, I removed it from this recipe. You may add ground flaxseed instead of oatmeal to make it smoother and creamier. I don't add any other spices, but you can add some cinnamon.

Add all ingredients together and let them boil. You can use a wooden spoon to smash and stir the ingredients until it gets creamy.

Enjoy this easy and quick breakfast.

Home-Made Almond Milk by Tsao-Lin Moy

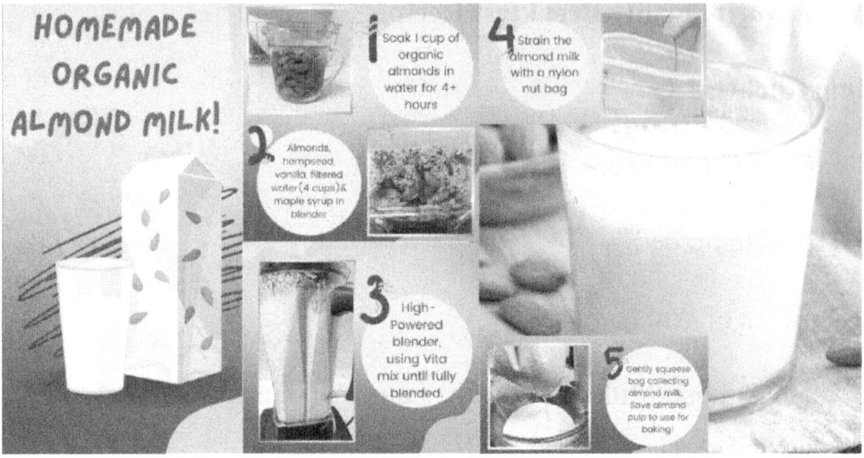

Step1: Soak 1 cup of organic almonds in water over 4 hours

Step2,3: Add almonds, hempseed, vanilla and 4 cups of filtered water in a blender until fully blended

Step 4: Gently squeeze bag collecting almond milk. You can save almond pulp for your baking purposes.

Turkey PHO Grain-free Noodle Soup by Heather Gray

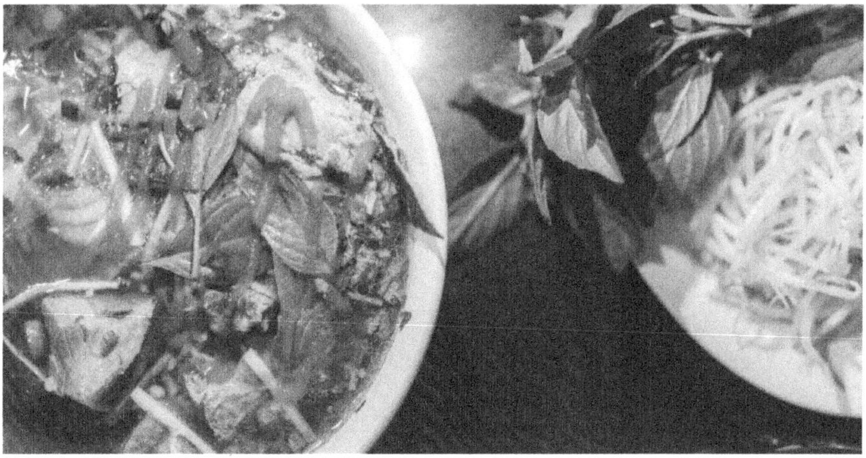

Ingredients

2 Tbsp. Avocado oil

3 Garlic cloves, pressed

1 Tbsp. fresh ginger, grated

3 Tbsp. Thai red curry paste

1 package ground organic turkey

5 c. chicken broth (turkey if you have it)

1 1/2 c. filtered water

2 1/2 Tbsp. fish sauce

1 can organic coconut milk

1 package of Miracle noodles (these are made from mushrooms), drained

1 package of mushrooms of your choice (washed and cut up)

For topping

1 lime cut into 4 quarters

Diced red onion

Red chili flakes

Cilantro

Mung bean sprouts

Radishes

Basil

In your Instant pot, use the Sautee feature and put in avocado oil. When hot, add the garlic, ginger, and curry paste. Sautee for a few minutes. Turn off the Sautee feature.

Sprinkle garlic salt, garlic powder, and paprika on the ground turkey, and form into 2 to 3-inch balls, place in the Instant pot.

Add all the other ingredients (except the toppings) into the Instant pot. Cook for 10 minutes. When the timer is done, do a quick release and serve. Make sure to put lots of your favorite toppings on top. YUM

Cinnamon Chia Seed Pudding and Breakfast Cookies by Kellie Lupsha

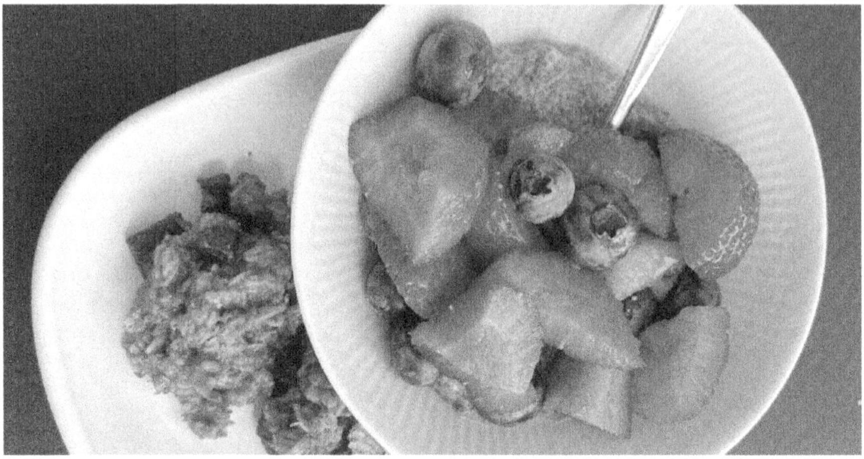

Loaded with protein, fiber, and Omega-3s. This is gluten free, paleo, and keto.

STEP ONE–Mix together in a glass bowl with a lid or glass mason jar. Stir/shake to break up any clumps. Let sit for 5 min and stir again.

- 3–4 Tbsp. chia seeds
- 1 c. Coconut Milk (or Almond Milk)
- ½ tsp. Cinnamon (for your taste)
- ¼ - ½ tsp. Vanilla

- 1 Tbsp. Sugar Substitute. I use monk fruit, erythritol, or stevia (again, modify per your taste)

STEP TWO - Put in the refrigerator overnight or for at least 2–3 hours.

STEP THREE–The chia seed pudding should be nice and thick. If it is still liquid, add 1 tsp–1 Tbsp. more of the chia seeds, stir and refrigerate for another 30 min.

- Add fresh seasonal fruit

- My favorite are berries: blueberries and strawberries.

Breakfast Cookies

Great for healthy options on the go. These are also gluten and dairy free. Wondering what to do with your overripe bananas besides banana bread? I've got you covered.

Preheat oven to 350 degrees Fahrenheit (175 degrees Celsius)

- 3 ripe bananas

- ½ c. almond butter (or other nut butter)

- 2 c. organic non-GMO rolled oats

- Mix in's.... I use ¼ c. dairy-free chocolate chips by Enjoy Life.

STEP ONE–Mash your bananas, put in a mixing bowl with almond butter and oats, and mix well. Add your mix in's. (You could add nuts, dried fruit, or even flax seed)

STEP TWO - Transfer cookies onto a lined baking sheet. The mixture will be quite moist, so to avoid sticking to your hands, either dampen hands before placing the cookies on the sheet or use a scooper. *My secret, I sprinkle a tiny bit of sea salt flakes on top.

STEP THREE–Bake at 350 degrees Fahrenheit or 175 Celsius for 10–12 minutes. And ENJOY!

Apple Sour Cherry Stew by Betty Khalili

This is my mother's favorite dish. Since I talked about my mom's health issue in my chapter, I love to share this recipe since it reminds me a good memory.

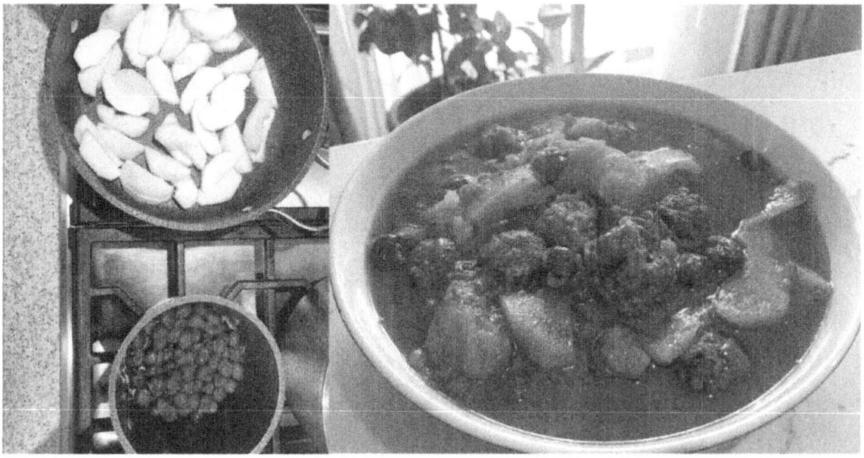

Ingredients (serving 4)

3 Tbsp. vegetable oil

1/4 tsp. ground saffron

2 Tbsp. salt

250g/8.8oz ground beef or lamb

2 big apples (Can be sour or sweet, depending on your taste)

5 Tbsp. vegetable oil

1/2 tsp. mild paprika

2 big onions

1/4 tsp. garlic powder

1/4 tsp. turmeric

1 lemon

1/4 tsp. black pepper

Method of Preparation

Marinate the meat

Shred one onion. Transfer the ground lamb or beef to a bowl, add paprika, shredded onion, turmeric, garlic powder, black pepper, and 1/4 tsp of salt.

Knead all the ingredients until they are well combined, and the spices are evenly distributed throughout the ground meat.

Cover the bowl with a plate so that the meat can firm a little before shaping the meatballs.

Shape the meatballs

Remove the ground meat from the fridge and oil a plate with some vegetable oil. This will prevent the meatballs from sticking to it, so you can let them slide into the pan.

Take a small amount of ground meat and shape a small ball by rolling it with both palms facing each other. The size I recommend going for is slightly larger than the sour cherries. The reason I make them so small is because I like them to be bitesize, so that you can have rice, as well as a sour cherry, and as a meatball on each spoon, without having to divide larger meatballs. Also, the small meatballs look better in this dish than chunky ones.

Transfer about 5 Tbsp. vegetable oil to a frying pan and put it over medium to high heat. If your frying pan is too small to fit all the meatballs and allows them to come in contact with the hot oil, divide them into two batches and use half the vegetable oil for each batch.

Once the oil is hot, add the meatballs to the pan and spread them out evenly. Since they are so small, you don't need to turn them individually. Gently shake the pan or give them a quick stir every minute or so, until they are golden brown all around. The whole process of searing them only takes about 5 minutes. Because of their small size, they may become tough and chewy if you leave them longer. Take them off the heat and transfer them to a bowl or plate.

Mix the stew ingredients

Wash and pit the sour cherries by cutting them hallway through. Add natural sweeteners like maple syrup or date syrup and stir them together.

Peel the green apples and slice them in wedges and sauté them in vegetable oil.

Squeeze lime on apples and mix well.

Add the ground saffron with a pinch of salt, pepper, and turmeric to sliced onion and fry them together.

Now you can add the meatballs, sour cherries, and sliced apples to the mix.

You can eat the stew with rice.

The dish in now ready to serve.

Good appetite!

Appendix - by Kellie Lupsha

Biological Pathways

Our bodies have many biochemical pathways that allow processes to occur. Pathways are made up of different proteins that work together in groups—similar to the way in which workers perform together on an assembly line.

"A biological pathway is a series of actions among molecules in a cell that leads to a certain product or a change in the cell. It can trigger the assembly of new molecules, such as a fat or protein, turn genes on and off, or spur a cell to move." **NIH, National Human Genome Research Institute.**

For your body to develop properly and stay healthy, many things must work together at many different levels - from organs to cells to genes.

From both inside and outside the body, cells are constantly receiving chemical cues prompted by such things as injury, infection, stress, or even the presence or lack of food. To react and adjust to these cues, cells send and receive signals through biological pathways. The molecules that make up biological pathways interact with signals, as well as with each other, to carry out their designated tasks. Biological pathways do not always work properly. When something goes wrong in a pathway, the result can be a disease such as cancer or diabetes. There are hundreds of these pathways that occur throughout the body, let's look a few that have recently become center stage in functional and longevity medicine.

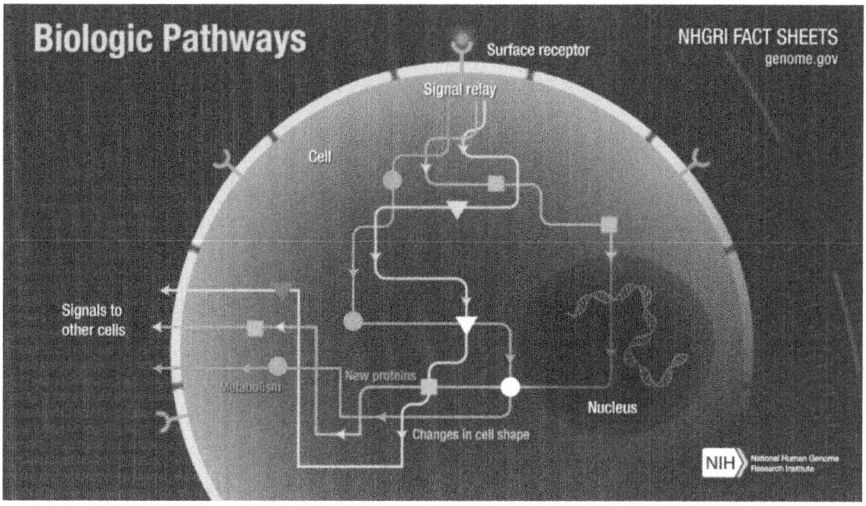

Figure2: Biologic Pathways

Nrf2 – Pathway

Nrf2 (nuclear factor erythroid-2-related factor 2) is a protein messenger that binds itself to DNA and is one of the master regulators of the body's aging process. The concept that Nrf2 is a

---

[30] Lewis KN, Mele J, Hayes JD, Buffenstein R. Nrf2, a guardian of healthspan and gatekeeper of species longevity. Integr Comp Biol 2010; 50: 829–843.

master regulator of not only longevity, but also more importantly, of health-span was suggested by Lewis *et al.* in their paper entitled "Nrf2, a guardian of health-span and gatekeeper of species longevity.[30]"

Nrf2 communicates with cells, instructing them to increase the number of active survival genes. Genes that allow the body to combat the effects from free radicals and other oxidants and help our bodies function at an optimal level. It goes into the nucleus of the cell and tells our DNA to produce proteins and enzymes. (See figure 1.) They can then get to work protecting and supporting the natural repair functions of our cells, mitochondria, and DNA from the inside. Hundreds of our genes, including many of our survival genes, are activated by Nrf2, including genes that are responsible for antioxidant response, detoxification, anti-inflammatory effects, cytoprotecting functions, and more. The cells adapt with both environmental and biological stresses less, which is typical as we age. This may seem overwhelming; let me simplify this process.

Free radicals are highly reactive and unstable molecules that are produced in the body naturally as a byproduct of normal metabolism, or by exposure to toxins in the environment such as tobacco smoke, ultraviolet light, pollution, and even our food and water and too much exercise, which cause damage to our cells. Oxidative stress is essentially an imbalance between the production of free radicals and the ability of the body to counteract or detoxify their harmful effects through neutralization by antioxidants. Think of oxidative stress as rusting of the cells. When you cut an apple and leave it out on the counter, over time it starts to turn brown. It oxidizes. This happens to every cell in the body as we age. Therefore, we must balance out the oxidants (bad guys) with antioxidants (good guys) to help optimize the body's ability to function.

This is what is so interesting about the Nrf2 protein verses direct antioxidants. When we take direct antioxidants like vitamin C, blueberries, or broccoli, what is happening inside our cells? We take antioxidants (good guys) to fight off free radicals (bad guys leading to cellular breakdown we call aging). When we eat our antioxidants, the body fight this battle of good guys to bad guys at a 1:1 ratio. Our bodies have trillions of free radicals (some references say we have a range between 1.3 – 2.4 sextillion or 10^{21}) so if we just fight the battle 1:1 with food and dietary antioxidants we may never win the battle. When you activate the Nrf2 protein, now your body is able to eliminate millions of free radicals per second, every second. This science is amazing; actually, our bodies are amazing. Now we start winning the battle in our bodies.

Washington State University said, "We may be on the verge of a new literature on health effects of Nrf2, which may well become the most extraordinary therapeutic and most extraordinary preventive breakthrough in the history of medicine. It is our opinion that raising

Nrf2 is likely to be the most important health promoting approach into the foreseeable future."

Nrf2, a master regulator of detoxification and also antioxidant, anti-inflammatory, and other cytoprotective mechanisms, is raised by health promoting factors[31].

Nrf2 was first discovered in 1992 and is gaining much popularity in the literature as we discover how to activate this protein. For the past several years, people have been using sulphoraphane (the active ingredients in broccoli and cauliflower) to turn on the Nrf2 pathway; however, research is exploding in this area with new products even more powerful at activating the Nrf2 pathway. You will see many Nrf2 activating products with combinations of ingredients using synergy, which are having powerful results. I highly suggest you begin activating this pathway to boost your longevity. As always, research the company and product before using, or even ask your practitioner for advice. You may find additional research on www.pubmed.gov Please understand you may not find many nutraceutical products in clinical research.

---

[31] *Acta Physiologica Sinica*, February 25, 2015, 67(1): 1–18 DOI: 10.13294/j.aps.2015.0001 http://www.actaps.com.cn

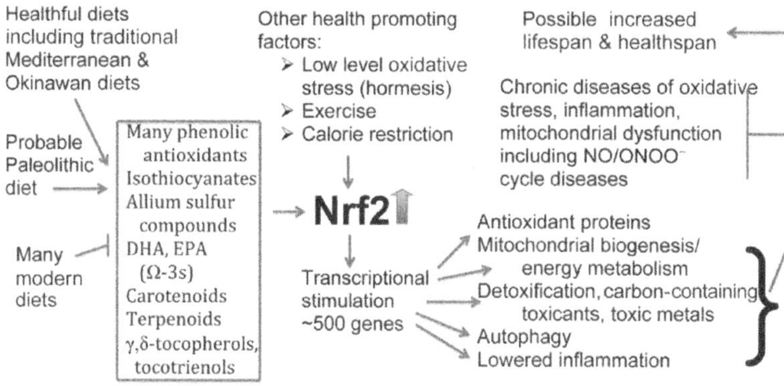

Fig. 3. Outline of the Nrf2 regulatory system[32].

Benefits of Activating the Nrf2 pathway

- Helps the body detoxify genes, keeping the master blueprint of the cell's function intact.
- Reduces oxidative stress.
- Significantly reduces cellular stress.
- Produces enzymes capable of neutralizing more than 1,000,000 free radicals.
- Help to regulate survival genes.

[32] Martin L Pall *et al.*: Nrf2, Master Cytoprotection & Detoxification Regulator, is Raised by Many Health Promoting Factors **11**

- Helps support healthy aging, that's been caused by oxidative stress.
- Enhance natural antioxidant production of SOD (Superoxide Dismutase), Catalase and Glutathione
- Promotes the cells' natural ability to repair and rejuvenate itself
- Protects cells from free radical damage

NRF1 Pathway

The NRF1 (nuclear factor erythroid 2-related factor 1) pathway is a major signaling pathway involved in mitochondrial health. Two main functions of NRF1 are to increase the biogenesis of mitochondria and to enhance autophagy (the body's way of cleaning out damaged cells in order to regenerate newer, healthier cells) to ensure healthy mitochondrial turnover. The NRF1 pathway stimulates an Nrf1 protein (Nuclear respiratory factor 1), which in turn activates key genes involved in metabolism, cellular growth, energy production, and mitochondrial DNA transcription and replication.

Mitochondria

The mitochondria[33] are part of a class of small subcellular compartments called organelles. All organelles have a specific function within the cell. So why are mitochondria so important? They make energy. They are essential to proper cellular function. Without functioning mitochondria, the cell has a significantly diminished capacity to generate or utilize energy for all its important metabolic processes. When they stop working, the cell stops working, and we stop working.

Their biggest job is to import nutrients, break them down, and turn them into complex molecules called ATP (Adenosine Triphosphate), the cell's battery pack. You may remember ATP from 7th grade biology. Tony Robbins calls mitochondria our Life Force Generators. Approximately 95% of the energy we need to function at any given moment in time is produced by the ever present and powerful mitochondria. The resultant energy molecule that the mitochondria produce for the cell is called ATP. Without ATP or the mitochondria that produce it, we would cease to exist.

The National Institute of Health funded a study that noted, "Perhaps no structure [mitochondria] is so intimately and simultaneously connected to both the energy of the youth and the

---

[33] Mitochondria: what are they and why are they important to my health? (mitoq.com)

decline of the old." * (Sun et al., "The Mitochondrial Basis of Aging.")

One of the things that many people don't realize is that in the process of breaking down food and converting it to energy, high energy electrons are generated. These electrons are usually captured by the mitochondria, where they harness their stored potential energy in a series of steps, and then ultimately bind to oxygen to form water and are rendered harmless. However, in the process of making ATP, some of these electrons are shed, and often escape being detoxified to oxygen and go on to create free radicals and other oxidants. As mitochondrial function declines over time-the conversion process becomes less efficient. Unfortunately, these metabolic by-products of energy formation (free radicals) contribute to mitochondrial decline. Thus, your mitochondria start to slow down and create an excess of free radicals and oxidative stress; the result is often widespread chronic inflammation throughout your body. Inflammation is a hot topic in the field of aging. Today, I'll just remind you that inflammation is the "Big Baddy" leading to many disease processes you don't want[34]!

[34] https://journals.physiology.org/doi/full/10.1152/physiol.00006.2017

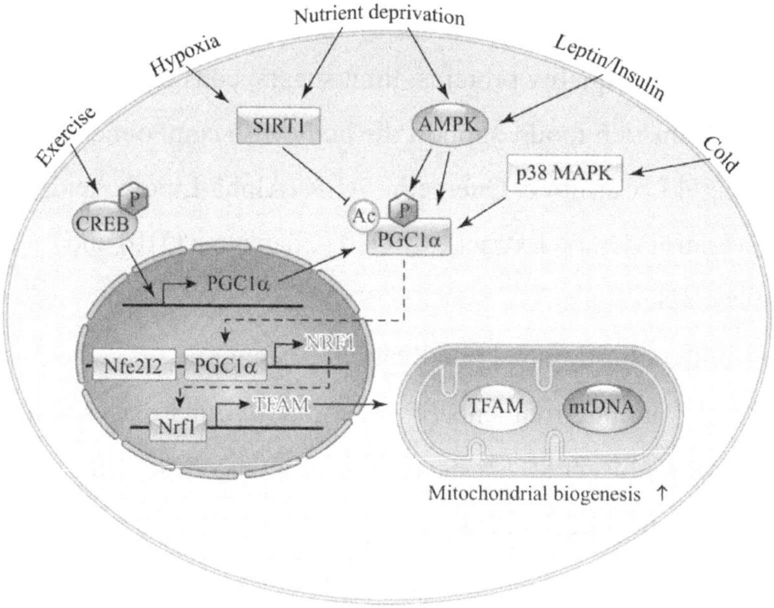

Fig. 4: Mitochondria[35]

Enhancing your Mitochondria

Choose from several of the following to enhance your energy

- Exercise, specifically HIIT (High Intensity Interval Training).
- Cold Therapy: Cryotherapy, ice baths, even ending your shower with 60 seconds of cold water).
- Heat Therapy: Infrared Sauna.
- Ozone Treatment.
- Sleep 7 – 8 hours in a cool and dark environment.
- Meditation: Decreases stress response and stress hormones.

[35] https://journals.physiology.org/doi/full/10.1152/physiol.00006.2017

- Food and Nutrition: Focus on burning fat for fuel, be mindful of eating high quality proteins, limit sugars, consume antioxidant-rich foods, support the body with compounds such as Acetyl L-Carnitine, Quercetin, ALA (Alpha-Lipoic Acid), Resveratrol (Grape Extract), CoQ10 (Coenzyme Q10) and Omega 3's.
- Intermittent Fasting or Time Restricted eating.
- * Check your environments (home, work, or other places you spend time) for mold, toxins, or heavy metals; these will damage your mitochondria.

What are Sirtuins and What is their Role in Longevity?

Sirtuins are a family of seven regulatory proteins that are critical epigenetic regulators. They sit at the top of the cellular system controlling our reproduction and our DNA repair. They also help govern our epigenome by turning on the right genes on and off at the right time, boosting mitochondrial activity, reducing inflammation, and protecting our telomeres. Now you are getting the idea of why they are so important in longevity. Dr. David Sinclair, in his book *Lifespan*, states, "Trading reproduction for repair, the sirtuins order our bodies to buckle down during times of stress and protect us against the major diseases of aging, like diabetes, heart disease, Alzheimer's disease, osteoporosis, and even cancer. They mute the chronic, overactive inflammation that drives diseases such as atherosclerosis, metabolic disorders, ulcerative colitis, arthritis, and asthma. They prevent cell death and boost mitochondria."

What is extremely important to understand is sirtuins require a molecule called NAD (Nicotinamide Adenine Dinucleotide). NAD powers the entire family of proteins. A sobering statistic to learn is we lose about half of our NAD+ around the age of 50. This puts us is a challenging situation because not only do our sirtuins have more work to do as we age, but they also don't have enough NAD+ fuel to do their job.

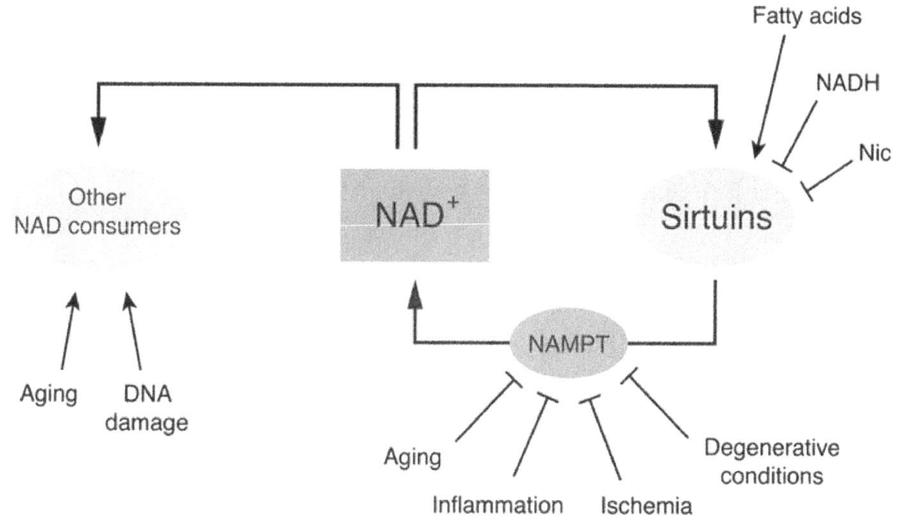

Figure 3: Regulation of the functional connection between NAD and sirtuins[36].

---

[36] https://www.researchgate.net/figure/Regulation-of-the-functional-connection-between-NAD-and-sirtuins-There-are-at-least_fig1_306312038

Thanks to Dr. Sinclair, lots of research is occurring today in the field of boosting NAD. There are several products on the market that are a precursor to NAD, boosting the body's sirtuins by 20 – 40%. However, new products are coming out that activate our own body's production of NAD and studies are showing levels increase anywhere from 100 – 300%. Current studies are underway that are being used by the US Special Forces. Today, this family of proteins, Sirtuins, is being coined as our Longevity Genes!

I want you to understand sirtuins deliver whole-body benefits, such as support for healthy longevity, the body's healthy inflammatory response, joint health, a healthy vascular system, and more. It even provides immediate benefits for energy, mood, and focus.

Supporting your Sirtuins

For now, here are several steps you can take to boost your sirtuin activity.

- Exercise, especially in HIIT (High Intensity Interval Training). Just FYI, you don't have to go to a class, you can stress your own body by lifting heavy weight, becoming breathless (get your HR, heart rate, to 70-85% of your max HR), in about 10 minutes to get this benefit. However, most of us need more accountability to get this done.

- Eat less and practice some form of intermittent fasting. (I suggest you consult with your practitioner before starting a fasting program).
- Just like boosting your mitochondria, build in a heat or cold exposure program. Exposing your body to less than comfortable temperatures is another great way to turn on these longevity genes.
- Find a product with a company you trust to activate your NAD.

Epilogue by Pantea Kalhor

Thank you so much for reading our book and allowing us to share our insights into integrative medicine and mind-body connection healing with you. I invited these specialists to help write this book so we can share our real case studies and give you true and practical information about how to recover from chronic pain and autoimmune disease. You cannot find this information through Google or in any other books.

The world suffers from so many chronic pain and autoimmune diseases these days that may lead to repetitive consumption of medications for a long period and create temporary relief from pain without searching for the actual root cause. This book is the professional evidence of how we can fill the gap between conventional and holistic medicine and how lifestyle can reverse most chronic diseases.

Some deaths can be easily avoided if we know how to find healing opportunities in our bodies and don't try to just remove our symptoms by taking pills. We can go deeper and look at the body as a whole. We also need to learn that our bodies, our minds, and our spirits are connected to each other, and so, treating the physical body demands an understanding of this binding.

I hope this book has helped you create a vision and plan for your future, a way out of the anxiety of suffering pain and torture that can come as a consequence of chronic pain or autoimmune disease. May you be armed with enough knowledge to continue with your healing journey.

If you have a story that can inspire others to rebuild their life again, please connect with me at http://acechoiceidea.com.

And don't forget to register in our landing page to receive your freebies and access our valuable masterclass.

http://acechoiceidea.com/funnel/needs-gap/

Pantea Kalhor

About the Authors

This book is collated and published by Pantea Kalhor and AceChoice Publishing and Branding.

Other authors are Reed Davis, Tsao-Lin Moy, Heather Gray, Kellie Lupsha, and Betty Khalili.

Pantea Kalhor

Publisher, Five Times Bestselling Author, Functional Nutrition Diagnostic Practitioner, Fertility Consultant, Show Host, and Podcaster

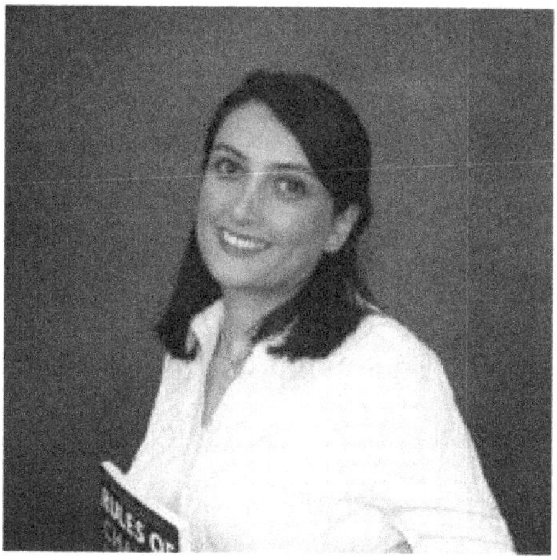

Pantea Kalhor

Pantea Kalhor is the author of five best-selling books: *The Gap Series, PTSD Compass*, *Naturally Conceived, Rules of Change for the Better,* and co-author of *Empowering Women to Succeed: Leap*. Her mission is to create a bridge between Western and Eastern medicine to show how holistic medicine and mind-body connection can help conventional medicine find underlying health issues which are usually ignored or left undiscovered.

After a car-hijacking accident when she was threatened at knifepoint, she started her journey of transformation and healing from PTSD (Post Traumatic Stress Disorder).

Years later, she wrote her first book, *Rules of Change for The Better*, describing her own personal stories of transition. Then she created "Transition by Pantea Kalhor," a podcast with interviews with healthcare and holistic medicine practitioners, medical doctors, functional medicine practitioners, and PTSD coaches. They share the message of hope and introduce different modalities in Post Trauma recovery and healing from chronic disease.

She is also a certified Functional Diagnostic Nutrition Practitioner (FDN) and fertility consultant. She helps couples who are struggling with fertility to have an optimistic result through functional labs and lifestyle change.

If you wish to share your message, become a bestselling author, or promote your own brand, you can contact Pantea through her website:

https://acechoiceidea.com

If you need to consult about your wellness or fertility issues, please visit her website here:

https://panteakalhor.com

If you suffer from chronic disease or PTSD and are in need of some empowerment, follow her on social media.

Facebook: https://www.facebook.com/panteakalhorcoach

Instagram: https://www.instagram.com/panteakalhorcoach

YouTube:
https://www.youtube.com/c/PanteaKalhorTransitionChannel

Podcast: https://panteakalhor.libsyn.com/

Reed Davis

Bestselling Author, Founder of FDN (Functional Diagnostic Nutrition) Certification Course, Board-certified Holistic Health Practitioner (HHP), and Expert in Functional Lab Testing and Natural Protocols

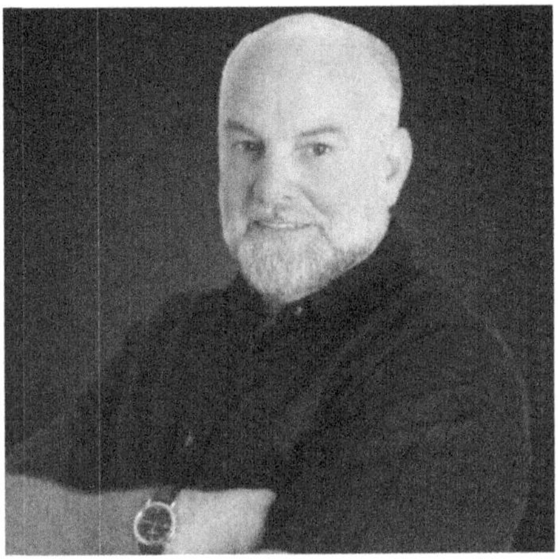

Reed Davis

Reed Davis is the Founder of FDN. He is a board-certified Holistic Health Practitioner (HHP) and expert in functional lab testing and natural protocols. He founded Functional Diagnostic Nutrition® (FDN) and the FDN Certification Course after serving as the case manager at a wellness center in Southern California for over ten years.

Having helped over 10,000 clients, Reed is known as one of the most experienced clinicians anywhere. He now serves on the

American Natural Wellness Coaches Advisory Board and the American Association of Natural Wellness Coaches. Reed lives in the U.S., teaching his course and helping graduates build their businesses, or may be found gardening or riding his motorcycle.

http://www.FDNthrive.com

Tsao-Lin Moy, Bestselling Author, Licensed Acupuncturist, Traditional Chinese Medicine Practitioner, and Herbalist

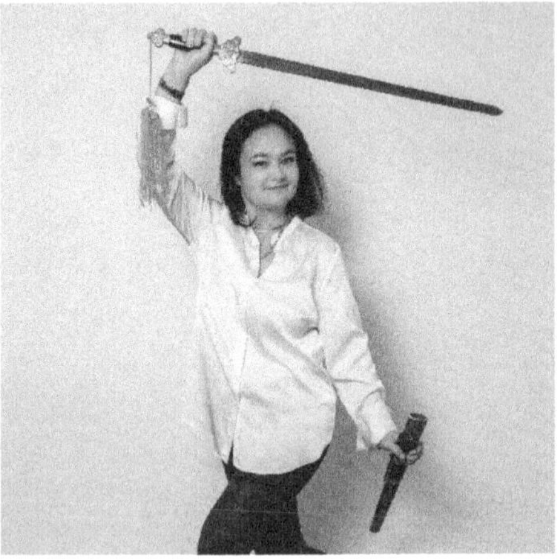

Tsao-Lin Moy

Tsao-Lin E. Moy is a natural fertility expert trained in East Asian medicine who helps couples conceive naturally using her fertility protocols and Chinese medicine. She is the founder of Integrative Healing Arts in NYC, which utilizes acupuncture, herbal medicine, and energy healing to treat patients.

Tsao has over 18 years of experience in alternative and Chinese medicine and is a licensed acupuncturist and herbalist. She is also the best-selling author of *Will I Ever Get Pregnant? The Smart Woman's Guide to Get Pregnant Naturally Over 40.*

https://www.integrativehealingarts.com/

https://www.instagram.com/tsaolinmoy

Heather Gray, FDN Practitioner, Lyme Boss

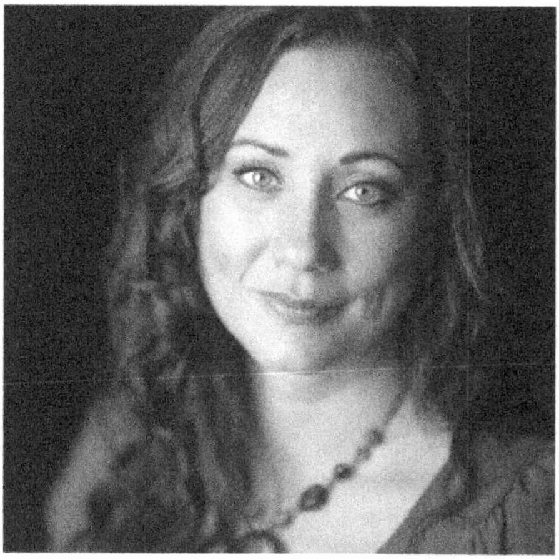

Heather Gray

Heather Gray is a Functional Diagnostic Nutritionist Practitioner. She found this work after 27 years of undiagnosed Lyme Disease, celiac disease, Hashimoto's, and endometriosis. She was depressed, anxious, and in chronic widespread pain, had bad skin, was bloated, constipated, exhausted, had weight gain, and had horrible periods, to name a few things. She set out on a path to healing. She has now lost over 100 pounds, her pain has lessened, she has no more suicidal thoughts, and has all-day energy. She now has a practice where she teaches others how to take care of themselves and get the inflammation off their body and brain. She gives you control over your health journey. She helps you destroy brain fog, moodiness, chronic inflammation, and pain.

Needs Gap

https://www.facebook.com/DiscoveringHealthFDN

https://www.instagram.com/heather_gray_lyme_boss/

https://www.youtube.com/channel/UCEh1w8d52wkr45ZOeAEWcOg

https://spotifyanchor-web.app.link/e/mOtGfUeIVub

https://www.discoveringhealthfdn.com

Kellie Lupsha, Women's Longevity Expert

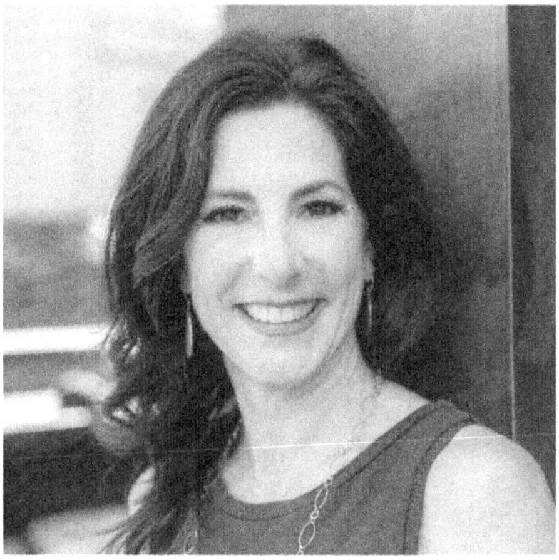

Kellie Lupsha

Kellie Lupsha is an expert on Women's Health in Energy and Longevity. She is foremost a mom of four kids and a true entrepreneur. Kellie has been in the wellness and healthcare space for 25 years. She has her Master's in Physical Therapy from the Mayo Clinic as well as a Master's in Business Management. Today, Kellie runs several online longevity programs, including a precision DNA and lifestyle program and an exclusive Mastermind for women over 40 looking to optimize their energy, focus, overall health, and life using the Vitality Method to live in abundant health! As a top priority, she is part of an international wellness company bringing a medical breakthrough in Nutrigenomics to the world. Her ultimate purpose is to elevate heath in the world and teach people to become the CEO of their own health! Learn more:

https://linktr.ee/kellielupsha

https://thelupshas.com

Contact her on messenger: Kellie Lupsha or info@thelupshas.com

Betty Khalili, Registered Nurse and Bestselling Author

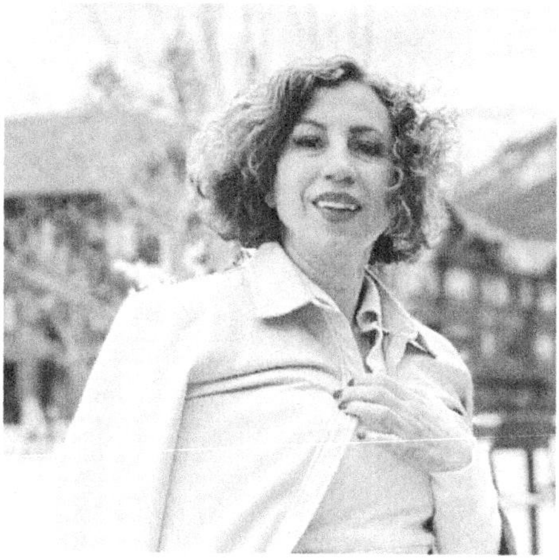

Betty Khalili

Betty Khalili is the best-selling author of "Not Simply Broken", Registered Nurse, Certified in Aesthetic sciences and the Life Coach. She Believes in Holistic Medicine and Lifestyle Changes. Successfully, she helped her mother heal from regurgitation attacks after 15 years of suffering. Betty helps her patients relieve from chronic pain by investigating their lifestyle and optimizing their health by simple modifications. Currently, she lives in Canada.

https://acechoiceidea.com/notsimplybroken/

https://www.instagram.com/nursebettytoronto/

Made in the USA
Monee, IL
04 November 2026

67383013R00105